AMERICAN COLLEGE OF PHYSICIANS

Healthy Heart
COOKBOOK

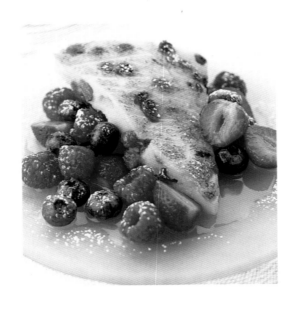

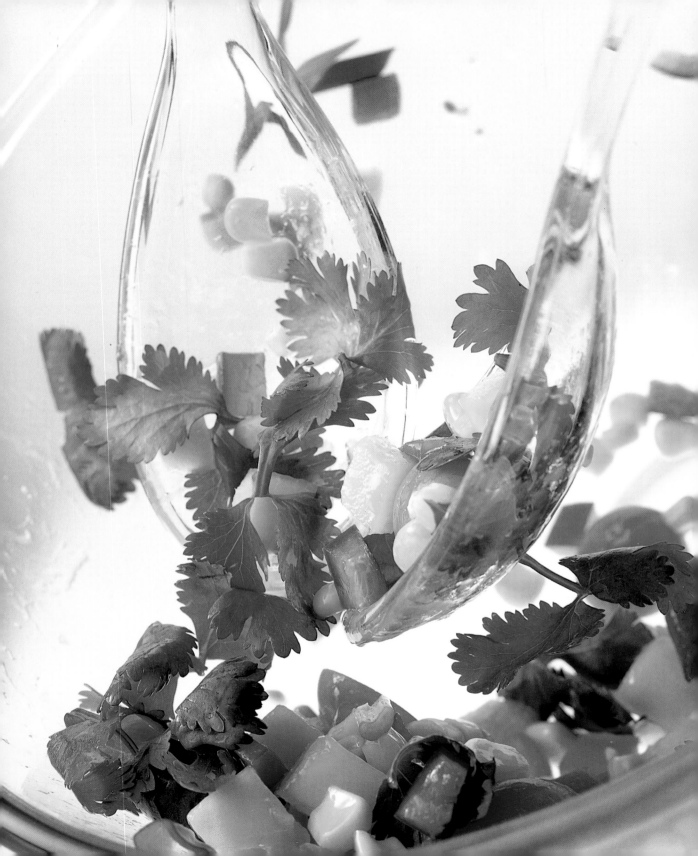

AMERICAN COLLEGE OF PHYSICIANS

Healthy Heart
COOKBOOK

Oded Schwartz

PHOTOGRAPHY IAN O'LEARY

FOOD STYLING JANE SUTHERING

MEDICAL EDITORS

LISA HARK, PhD, RD DAVID R. GOLDMANN, MD

FRANCES BURKE, MS RD

A Dorling Kindersley Book

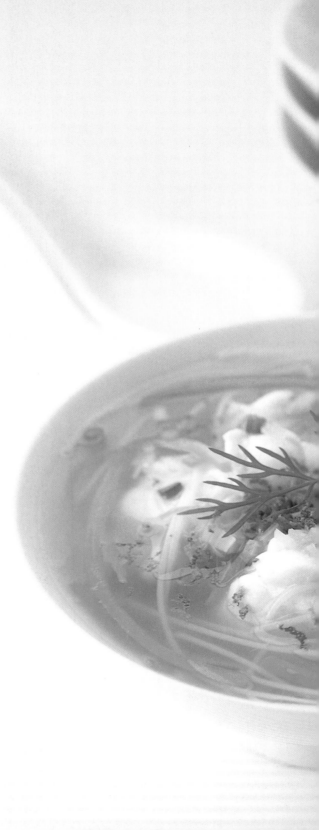

Dorling 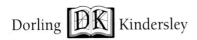 Kindersley

LONDON, NEW YORK, SYDNEY, DELHI, PARIS,
MUNICH, and JOHANNESBURG

Project Editors Nicola Graimes, Barbara Minton
Art Editor Sue Storey
Senior Editors Jude Garlick, Jill Hamilton
Senior Managing Editor Krystyna Mayer
Deputy Art Director Carole Ash
DTP Designer Conrad van Dyk
Production Controller Joanna Bull

Text for Nutrition & the Heart Luci Daniels, Lisa Hark

First published in the United States in 2000 by
Dorling Kindersley Publishing, Inc.
95 Madison Avenue, New York, New York 10016

Library of Congress Cataloging-in-Publication Data
Schwartz, Oded.
  Healthy heart cookbook / Oded Schwartz.
    p. cm.   Includes index.
  ISBN 0-7894-5176-X (alk. paper)
    1. Heart--Diseases--Diet therapy. 2. Low-fat diet--Recipes.
I. Title.
RC684.D5 S37 2000
616.1 20654--DC21
                                    99-086091

Reproduced in Italy by GRB Editrice, Verona
Printed and bound in China by L. Rex Printing Co. Ltd.

Recipe Points to Remember
All spoon measures are level unless otherwise stated
(1 teaspoon = 5ml, 1 tablespoon = 15ml). Eggs are medium.
Follow either imperial or metric measurements, never mix the
two. Baking times are a guide only, because every oven varies.

**Material in this book was reviewed by the ACP–ASIM for
general medical accuracy and applicability in the United
States; however, the information provided herein does not
necessarily reflect the specific recommendations or opinions
of the ACP–ASIM. The naming of an organization, product,
or alternative therapy in this book is not an ACP–ASIM
endorsement, and the omission of any such name does
not indicate ACP–ASIM disapproval.**

See our complete catalog at
www.dk.com

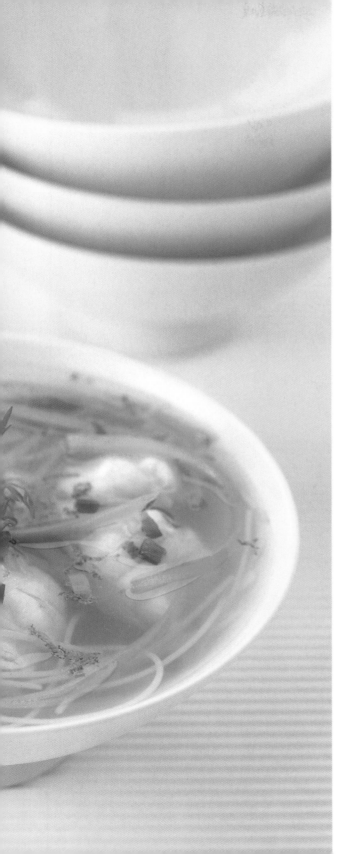

CONTENTS

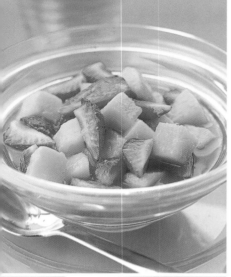

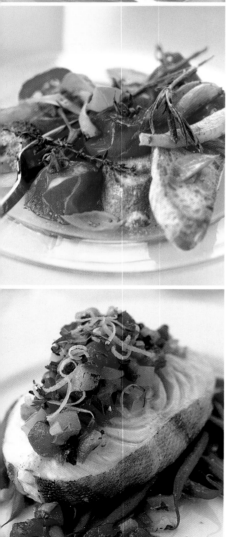

FOREWORD

Despite new medications and life-saving surgical procedures, heart disease still remains one of the most common killers in the developed world. Although our genetic makeup exerts significant influence on our health, several major modifiable lifestyle factors increase the risk of heart disease – and particularly coronary artery disease. Prevention of heart disease and treatment of three of the four major conditions that underlie it – high blood pressure, elevated levels of cholesterol, diabetes, and cigarette smoking – begin with changes in diet and physical activity.

The *American College of Physicians Healthy Heart Cookbook* starts with the premise that eating right is not only essential to prevention of heart disease but can also please the palate. The introductory material in the book enables you to understand the basic mechanisms underlying heart disease and to assess your own individual risk of developing it. Most important, it provides clear information on the basic constituents of diet and how each influences risk for heart disease. It offers simple guide-lines for losing excess weight, practical advice on choosing the right foods, and easy ways to modify recipes without sacrificing good taste.

The *Health Heart Cookbook* contains more than 100 recipes for all occasions, from a quick, nutritious breakfast to an elegant dinner for friends or family. Even those people with limited time available for cooking will find a wide variety of imaginative brunch choices, entrees, salads, side dishes, and delicious desserts. Each recipe has been carefully crafted to provide the right balance of nutrients and extensively taste-tested. So take control of your health by starting today. Heart-healthy food has never tasted so good!

LISA HARK, PhD, RD, AND DAVID R. GOLDMANN, MD, FACP
AMERICAN COLLEGE OF PHYSICIANS–AMERICAN SOCIETY OF INTERNAL MEDICINE

INTRODUCTION

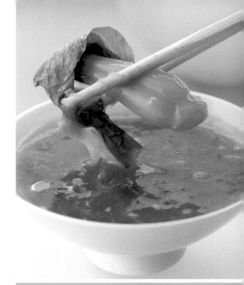

Having a heart problem does not mean that you have to give up all your favorite foods. As the recipes in this book will verify, producing inspiring, fresh, low fat and low sodium dishes can be just as easy and creative as any other style of cooking.

Often all that is required is a little more thought, planning, and patience to train your palate to enjoy a wide range of foods that provide different and tantalizing new flavors and textures. Instead of limiting what you can eat, the following recipes allow you to broaden your options, and encourage the use of many varied ingredients.

For some people, the recipes will offer a radical change in eating habits. Care has been taken to ensure that the recipes are low both in salt and fat, and fresh herbs, spices, lemon juice, vinegar, and mustard have been used extensively to give flavor and texture.

Meeting the demands for and interest in contemporary, fusion-style dishes, the recipes draw inspiration from the diverse culinary traditions of the Mediterranean, the Middle East, India, and Southeast Asia – areas that have produced some of the healthiest cuisines in the world.

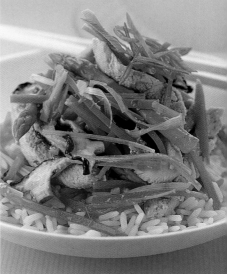

ODED SCHWARTZ

Nutritional Information

The recipes in this book are accompanied by detailed nutritional analyses of calories, carbohydrate, protein, fat, fiber, cholesterol, and sodium. The figures are based on data from food composition tables, with additional information about manufactured products. Ingredients that are described as "optional" are not included in the nutritional analyses. For further information, see page 128.

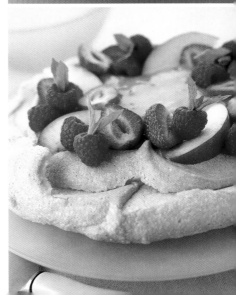

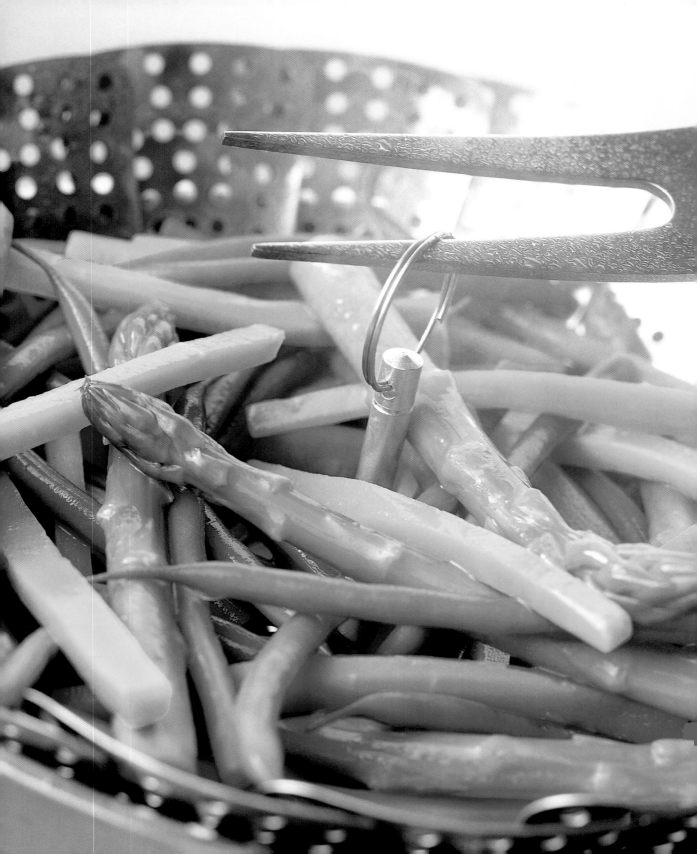

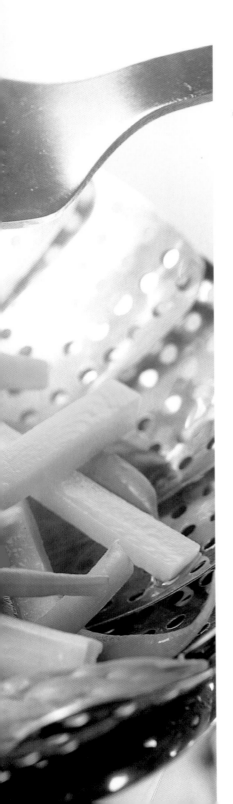

NUTRITION & THE HEART

THIS CHAPTER CONTAINS POSITIVE AND *helpful* ADVICE THAT ENABLES YOU TO ENJOY A NUTRITIOUS DIET AND *healthy lifestyle*, WHICH ARE IMPORTANT FACTORS IN LIMITING THE RISK OF HEART DISEASE. ACHIEVING THE *right balance* FOR GOOD HEALTH IS *made easy* WITH GUIDELINES FOR *meal planning* AND STEP-BY-STEP PHOTOGRAPHS OF *key* COOKING TECHNIQUES.

UNDERSTANDING HEART DISEASE

DURING THE LAST TWENTY YEARS, SCREENING, EARLY DETECTION, AND ASSESSING THE RISK OF HEART DISEASE HAVE BECOME A MAJOR PRIORITY OF THE MEDICAL PROFESSION. IMPROVED NUTRITION AND ADVANCES IN MEDICAL TREATMENT HAVE REDUCED THE NUMBER OF DEATHS BUT HEART DISEASE STILL REMAINS THE MOST COMMON CAUSE OF DEATH IN DEVELOPED COUNTRIES.

THE RISKS ASSOCIATED WITH HEART DISEASE

The risk factors linked with heart disease can be divided into two distinct groups: non-modifiable factors, which are largely predetermined, and modifiable factors – those that can be directly influenced by lifestyle.

Non-modifiable factors
- Age: men over 45 and women over 55.
- Gender: incidence of heart disease is higher in men than in premenopausal women.
- Heredity: the risk of a heart attack is greater if there is a family history of premature heart disease.

Modifiable factors
- High cholesterol levels.
- High LDL levels.
- Low HDL levels.
- Current cigarette smoking.
- High blood pressure.
- Diabetes.
- Obesity.

Source: National Heart, Lung, and Blood Institute, National Cholesterol Education Program (NCEP).

What is heart disease? This general term describes any condition that affects the heart's ability to pump blood. "Cardiovascular disease" includes disease of the heart or of the arteries and veins making up the circulatory system.

- **Coronary artery disease** occurs when the arteries bringing oxygen-rich blood to the heart become narrowed by a fatty substance called plaque. This buildup of plaque, known as atherosclerosis, can progressively restrict blood flow to the heart.

- **Angina** is chest pain that occurs when the heart does not receive enough oxygenated blood due to the partial narrowing of the coronary arteries, and is typically triggered by exercise or stress.

- **A heart attack** (also called a myocardial infarction) occurs when a blood clot forms on atherosclerotic plaque that has accumulated in a coronary artery and completely blocks the artery.

- **A stroke or cerebrovascular accident (CVA)** can be caused by a blood clot in the blood vessels that supply the brain or by a hemorrhage in the brain.

- **Hyperlipidemia** refers to an elevated blood cholesterol or triglyceride level, and is most commonly associated with atherosclerosis. Lowering blood cholesterol levels can reduce the number of first and recurrent heart attacks, strokes, and cardiac deaths.

- **Low-density lipoprotein (LDL)** is one of several proteins in the blood that carry cholesterol in the blood to the tissues and organs. It is often referred to as the "bad cholesterol" since high levels are associated with an increased risk of heart disease.

- **High-density lipoprotein (HDL)** is the protein in the blood that carries cholesterol from the tissues back to the liver. It is often referred to as the "good cholesterol" since high levels are associated with a reduced risk of heart disease.

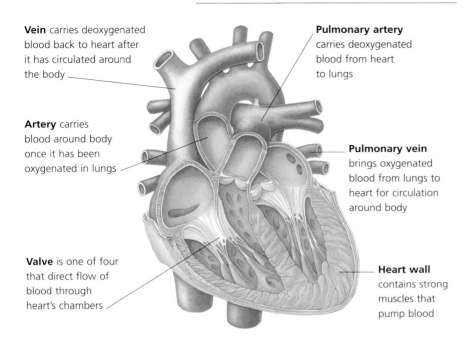

Vein carries deoxygenated blood back to heart after it has circulated around the body

Artery carries blood around body once it has been oxygenated in lungs

Valve is one of four that direct flow of blood through heart's chambers

Pulmonary artery carries deoxygenated blood from heart to lungs

Pulmonary vein brings oxygenated blood from lungs to heart for circulation around body

Heart wall contains strong muscles that pump blood

HOW THE HEART WORKS
The heart is a powerful muscle that functions as two coordinated pumps. One sends blood to the lungs to pick up oxygen, then the other pumps oxygenated blood throughout the body. Four chambers and four valves control the flow of blood. Problems are most often due to disruption of the pumping action of the heart because narrowing of the arteries decreases the supply of oxygenated blood to the heart muscle.

Assessing your risk

High blood cholesterol and LDL levels, low HDL levels, smoking, high blood pressure, and diabetes are all modifiable risk factors over which we have control. Here are the important facts and their relation to diet and lifestyle.

- **Total cholesterol levels**: An elevated blood cholesterol level, usually greater than 200 mg/dL, may be inherited or influenced by dietary factors, specifically a diet that is high in both total and saturated fat.

- **LDL levels**: High LDL levels reflect hereditary factors as well as high saturated fat intake. LDL target goals are based upon an individual's risk status (see opposite). If LDL levels are not responsive to diet and exercise therapy, drug therapy should be initiated.

- **HDL levels** below 35 mg/dL for men, 45 mg/dL for women, are considered a risk factor for heart disease. Lifestyle changes, such as weight loss, exercise, and smoking cessation, increase HDL levels.

- **Smoking** increases the risk of heart disease by increasing LDL and decreasing HDL levels. Continuing to smoke after a heart attack doubles the risk of a future attack.

- **High blood pressure** (hypertension), defined as greater than 140/90mmHg, tends to run in families. In addition to medication, lifestyle changes such as weight loss, exercise, decreasing dietary sodium, and limiting alcohol intake are helpful in treating high blood pressure.

- **Diabetes** increases the risk of heart disease more than four-fold. Normalizing blood sugar levels by means of diet, exercise, and medication is critical to reducing complications associated with diabetes.

- **Obesity** Losing a modest amount of excess weight can help reduce LDL levels, blood pressure, and the risk of heart disease. Use the chart on page 13 to assess your weight. Lose weight gradually by decreasing your calorie intake and increasing your activity level. A reduction of 500 calories every day will enable you to lose one pound per week.

HEART DISEASE & DIET

THERE IS STRONG EVIDENCE TO SUGGEST A LINK BETWEEN THE FOODS WE
EAT AND THE RISK OF DEVELOPING HEART DISEASE. A HEART-HEALTHY DIET SHOULD
CONTAIN A MODEST AMOUNT OF FAT AND SALT, WITH PLENTY OF FRUIT AND
VEGETABLES FOR FIBER AND ANTIOXIDANTS.

**TARGET DAILY INTAKES OF
TOTAL FAT AND SATURATED
FAT ACCORDING TO
CALORIE LEVEL**

Total fat recommendations
are calculated at 30% of
total calories and saturated
fat at 10% of total calories,
according to the NCEP
Step One diet.

Here are some examples
○ 1500 calories
50 grams of fat
17 grams saturated fat

○ 2000 calories
67 grams of fat
22 grams saturated fat

○ 2500 calories
83 grams of fat
28 grams saturated fat

Protective foods

Numerous studies have confirmed that certain foods may have a positive effect on the heart and should form the foundation of a healthy diet.

● **Fruits and vegetables** are excellent sources of vitamins, minerals, and other antioxidants (*see page 17*), which have been shown to reduce the risk of heart disease by supporting the body's defense system. They may also help to prevent the "furring up" of the arteries to the heart. Fruits and vegetables also provide soluble fiber and folic acid, a vitamin known to reduce levels of the amino acid homocysteine in the blood. High homocysteine levels have been found to increase the risk of developing heart disease, and research is under way to establish whether eating greater amounts of foods containing folic acid may help to reduce the risk of heart disease.

● **Oily fish** such as herring, salmon, mackerel, and sardines are good sources of omega-3 fatty acids, which have been found to reduce the likelihood of blood clots and to lower levels of cholesterol in the blood.

● **Oatmeal, beans, lentils, and nuts** are good sources of soluble fiber, which can help to lower blood-cholesterol levels (*see page 17*).

Non-protective foods

It is important to reduce the amount of non-protective foods included the diet since these can increase the risk of heart disease.

● **Fat**, particularly saturated fat (*see page 16*), has been linked to high blood-cholesterol levels and obesity. High fat consumption and a low intake of protective foods (*see above*) increases the risk of heart disease.

● **Salt** can cause an increase in blood pressure and should be eaten only in moderation (*see page 17*).

Weight distribution

Studies have shown that the distribution of body fat in overweight people also influences the risk of heart disease.

● "Apple-shaped" people carry any excess fat around their waist, which increases the pressure on the heart. It is this pattern of weight distribution that is most commonly associated with heart disease, increased cholesterol levels, and diabetes.

● "Pear-shaped" people have excess fat around the hips, bottom, and thighs and have a lower risk of developing heart disease than those with an apple shape.

Weight control

Being overweight causes an increase in both cholesterol levels and blood pressure. Weight control is an important factor in looking after the health of the heart, and losing even a modest amount of excess weight can help reduce these levels. Use the chart below to assess your weight. If it indicates that you need to lose weight, set realistic goals and aim to lose weight gradually. Weight-reducing diets are more effective when combined with regular physical activity.

WEIGHT-LOSS GUIDELINES

Those wishing to lose weight should reduce both calorie and fat intakes. Follow the lesser figure given in the guidelines if you are not very active, and the greater figure if you are able to increase your level of activity.

Weight-loss diet for men
❍ 1500–1800 calories a day
❍ 50–60g fat, of which no more than 15–20g should be saturated fat.

Weight-loss diet for women
❍ 1200–1500 calories a day
❍ 40–50g fat, of which no more than 12–15g should be saturated fat.

BODY MASS INDEX CHART

To assess your weight, follow a straight line across from your height (without shoes) and a line up from your weight (without clothes). Put a mark where the two lines meet.

KEY TO CHART
Underweight You may need to eat more, but choose nutritious foods (see p.17). If you are severely underweight, see your doctor.
Normal weight You are keeping your weight at a desirable level, but make sure your diet is healthy.
Overweight It would be beneficial to your health to lose some

weight and prevent additional weight gain.
Obese It is important to lose weight since your health may be at risk. It is advisable to see your doctor or dietitian and lose weight.
Severely Obese Being this overweight could be a serious risk to your health. It is important to see your doctor or a dietitian and lose weight.

HEIGHT

Metres	Feet
1.9m	6ft 3in
1.88m	6ft 2in
1.89m	6ft 1in
1.83m	6ft
1.8m	5ft 11in
1.78m	5ft 10in
1.75m	5ft 9in
1.73m	5ft 8in
1.70m	5ft 7in
1.68m	5ft 6in
1.65m	5ft 5in
1.63m	5ft 4in
1.6m	5ft 3in
1.58m	5ft 2in
1.55m	5ft 1in
1.52m	5ft
1.5m	4ft 11in
1.47m	4ft 10in

Lbs: 84, 98, 112, 126, 140, 154, 168, 182, 196, 210, 224, 238, 252, 266, 280, 294, 308, 322, 350

WEIGHT

Kg: 38, 44.5, 51, 57, 63.5, 70, 76, 83, 89, 95.5, 102, 108, 114.5, 121, 127, 133.5, 140, 146, 153, 159

GETTING THE RIGHT BALANCE

MEETING YOUR DAILY DIETARY REQUIREMENTS FOR OPTIMAL HEALTH IS EASY USING THE FOLOWING

PIE CHART. IT IS IMPORTANT TO EAT A VARIED DIET AND TO CHOOSE FOODS FROM THE MAIN

FOOD GROUPS BECAUSE NO SINGLE FOOD CAN SUPPLY ALL OUR NUTRITIONAL NEEDS.

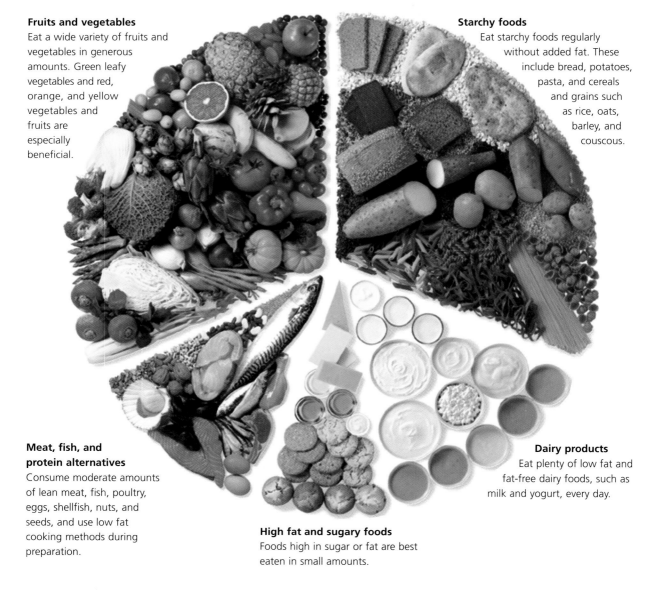

Fruits and vegetables
Eat a wide variety of fruits and vegetables in generous amounts. Green leafy vegetables and red, orange, and yellow vegetables and fruits are especially beneficial.

Starchy foods
Eat starchy foods regularly without added fat. These include bread, potatoes, pasta, and cereals and grains such as rice, oats, barley, and couscous.

Meat, fish, and protein alternatives
Consume moderate amounts of lean meat, fish, poultry, eggs, shellfish, nuts, and seeds, and use low fat cooking methods during preparation.

High fat and sugary foods
Foods high in sugar or fat are best eaten in small amounts.

Dairy products
Eat plenty of low fat and fat-free dairy foods, such as milk and yogurt, every day.

- **Starchy foods** At least one-third of what we eat, or about six servings a day, should include potatoes, bread, rice, pasta, whole grains, and breakfast cereals. One serving is equivalent to a medium baked potato, a small sweet potato, a small bowl of cooked rice, pasta, or cereal, or one slice of bread. Starchy foods, especially unrefined versions, are naturally low in fat and are usually high in B vitamins, minerals, and dietary fiber. Be careful to avoid adding butter, cheese, or cream sauce to these foods during preparation.

- **Fruit and vegetables** Eat at least five servings a day. Fresh, frozen, or dried, fruits and vegetables are an excellent source of vitamins, minerals, fiber, and valuable antioxidants. One serving is equivalent to a medium-sized fruit, a half of a banana, four ounces of fruit juice, or a half-cup of vegetables. Avoid creamy vegetable soups and vegetables that are prepared in butter or served with cream sauces, which add excess saturated fat.

- **Dairy products** Eat at least three servings a day. Dairy products are a good source of protein, vitamins, and minerals, especially calcium, which is essential for healthy bones and teeth. It is important to choose low fat dairy products since whole milk brands are high in saturated fat. The following are equivalent to one serving: 8 oz. of fat-free or 1% milk or 8oz. of fat-free or low fat yogurt. Substituting evaporated skim milk for cream in soups and other recipes will provide the creaminess without the added fat.

- **Meat, poultry, and protein alternatives** Eat less than 6 to 8 oz. a day. Try to aim for more vegetarian meals, such as chickpeas, pastas, bean, or lentils dishes that we have developed. When preparing meat or poultry, be sure to remove excess fat before cooking, and grill, steam, bake, or broil so that the fat can drip down into the pan. The white meat of turkey and chicken, without the skin, is significantly lower in fat than the dark meat.

- **Fish and shellfish** are an excellent alternative to meat and poultry because of their low total fat and saturated fat content. The cholesterol content of shellfish varies, but, if they are steamed, broiled or grilled without adding fat, it can be included frequently in a heart healthy diet.

- **High fat and sugary foods** Limit intake of cakes, candies, pastries, potato chips, chocolate, ice cream, creamy soups, and sauces. They are high in saturated fat and easily contribute to eight gain. Choose fruits and vegetables for nutritious snacks.

DRINKING MORE WATER

Try to drink at least eight glasses of water every day to maintain hydration.

○ Since caffeinated drinks and alcohol can contribute to dehydration and sweetened drinks, such as iced teas, colas, and juices, contribute excess calories, water or herbal teas makethe best choices.

ALCOHOL

Alcohol need not be entirely excluded from a heart healthy diet unless your doctor has advised you not to drink. However, moderation is the key; drinking too much can negatively effect your health by increasing your blood pressure or damaging your liver and pancreas. Moderate alcohol intake is defined as no more than two drinks per day for women and no more than three per day for men.

One unit of alcohol is equivalent to:
○ 11fl oz beer
○ 4½ fl oz wine
○ 1½ fl oz hard liquor

FACTS ABOUT FOOD

FOOD CHOICES AND EATING HABITS ARE IMPORTANT FACTORS IN HELPING PEOPLE WITH HEART DISEASE.

A HEALTHY HEART DIET SHOULD CONTAIN A MODEST AMOUNT OF FAT WITH PLENTY OF STARCHY

FOODS AND FRUITS AND VEGETABLES. IT IS ALSO IMPORTANT TO MODIFY SALT INTAKE AND TO

ENSURE REGULAR INTAKES OF FIBER AND ANTIOXIDANT NUTRIENTS.

SOURCES OF SATURATED FATS

○ Meats/Poultry: brisket, corned beef, regular ground beef, sausages, hot dogs, bacon, luncheon meats, pâté, spare ribs, lamb, lard, and poultry skin.

○ Dairy products: butter, whole milk, 2% milk, heavy cream, half-n-half, whipped cream, full-fat yogurt and cottage cheese, ice cream, hard cheeses, and regular cream cheese.

○ Breads/Snacks: potato chips, croissants, butter or sweet rolls, quick breads, and biscuits.

○ Desserts/Sweets: donuts, cakes, candy, pies, Danish, pastries, and cookies.

Fats The National Cholesterol Education Program (NCEP) issued recommendations in 1987 and 1993 to guide management of high blood cholesterol levels in adults. Dietary modification is the cornerstone of management for all individuals with high LDL levels regardless of whether they require drug therapy or not. Lowering LDL levels may require significant lifestyle adjustments that are best accomplished gradually over time.

● **Saturated fats** A diet that is high in saturated fats has been linked to high LDL levels and heart disease. Reducing saturated fat to less than 8–10 percent of total caloric intake is recommended. Saturated fats are found mainly in meats, dairy products, processed snacks, and desserts (see left). Always choose small helpings of lean meat and limit your intake of fatty meats, full-fat dairy products, and desserts.

● **Monounsaturated fats** Diets rich in monounsaturated fats, such as those eaten by people living in countries of the Mediterranean region, are associated with a lower incidence of heart disease. Olive oil, canola oil, rapeseed oil, sesame oil, peanuts, and avocados are high in monounsaturated fats and should be the predominant sources of fat in the diet. Monounsaturated fats can represent up to 15 percent of total calories.

● **Polyunsaturated fats** There are two categories of polyunsaturated fats: omega-3 fatty acids and omega-6 fatty acids. Oily fish, such as tuna, salmon, Chilean sea bass, herring, mackerel, and sardines, are high in omega-3 fatty acids, and have been found to reduce the likelihood of blood clots forming and also to lower blood pressure and blood triglyceride levels. Eat grilled or broiled fish at least once per week. Omega-6 fatty acids are found in vegetable oils such as sunflower oil, corn oil, safflower oil, and soybean oil. They are essential for growth, maintaining cell structure, a healthy immune system, and the regulation of blood. Polyunsaturated fats can represent up to 10 percent of total calories.

● **Trans fatty acids** Also known as hydrogenated fats, trans fatty acids are found in some cooking fats, margarine, pastries, cookies, and prepared foods. They act like saturated fats to increase LDL levels. Since many food manufacturers are cutting down on the use of hydrogenated fats, always check ingredients lists for "partially hydrogenated" oils.

Cholesterol

Egg yolks, fish roe, liver, and other organ meats contain the highest amounts of dietary cholesterol; however, it has been found that dietary saturated fat intake has a greater impact on total and LDL levels than dietary cholesterol alone. For example, although shrimp has a moderate amount of cholesterol, its saturated fat content is so low that it can be included in a heart healthy diet. The NCEP recommends limiting dietary cholesterol to less than 300mg/day.

Salt

High salt intake has been linked to heart disease, high blood pressure, and stroke. Consequently, controlling salt intake is an important part of a heart healthy diet. Cutting down on high salt foods is essential (see right). Season food with pepper, fresh or dried herbs, spices, lemon juice, vinegar, or mustard. In general, foods with more than 500mg of salt per serving are considered high in salt content.

Fiber

There are two types of dietary fiber – insoluble and soluble. Soluble fiber is found in vegetables, fruits, beans, oats, and lentils, and can help reduce blood cholesterol levels. Insoluble fiber, found in whole grains and bran, has no effect on blood cholesterol but helps prevent constipation. Fiber intake should total 30–40 g/day.

Antioxidants

Free radicals are chemical compounds in the body that can damage and cause narrowing of the arteries. Antioxidants may help prevent this. The main antioxidants are vitamins A (as beta-carotene), C, and E and selenium, zinc, copper, and manganese. Fruits and vegetables are excellent sources of antioxidants.

Folic Acid

High levels of the amino acid homocysteine have been found to increase the risk of developing heart disease and can be reduced by eating more folic acid. Folic acid is found in dark-green leafy vegetables, whole-grain cereals, beans, oranges, orange juice, and fortified breakfast cereals.

LOW FAT TIPS

○ Avoid fried foods, creamy soups and sauces, high-fat snacks, pastries, and cakes.

○ Broil, roast, bake, steam, or microwave food with small amounts of unsaturated fat.

○ Steam or boil vegetables and do not smother them after cooking with butter, margarine, or rich sauces.

○ Use small amounts of low fat spreads and salad dressings that are based on unsaturated fats.

SOURCES OF HIGH SALT CONTENT

○ Packaged or prepared frozen meals.

○ Canned foods such as soups, tuna fish, and tomato products.

○ Smoked or salted meats and fish such as lox, herring, and kippered salmon.

○ Meats: bacon, hot dogs, salt pork, scrapple, and most cold cuts.

○ Snacks (salted) such as potato chips, pretzels, peanuts, and popcorn.

○ Condiments such as soy sauce, barbecue sauce, relish, meat tenderizers, pickles, olives, sauerkraut, and bouillon cubes.

Buying & Cooking Food

READING THE LABELS ON PACKAGED FOODS, WHICH HAVE BEEN STANDARDIZED BY THE UNITED STATES FOOD AND DRUG ADMINISTRATION, PROVIDES INFORMATION THAT WILL HELP YOU MAKE HEALTHY CHOICES. SINCE THE NUTRITIONAL VALUES GIVEN ARE THE AMOUNT PER 100G, YOU SHOULD ALWAYS NOTE THE SERVING SIZE WHEN YOU ARE COMPARING THE NUTRITIONAL CONTENT OF FOOD PRODUCTS.

What the labels say When reading the nutritional information given on a food label, concentrate on the figures for the total fat and saturated fat content. To achieve a total fat intake of less than 30 percent, try to eat those foods that contain less than 30 percent fat calories. The number of fat calories is listed directly next to total calories on a food label (see below). You can determine the percentage of fat calories by dividing the number of fat calories by the total calories figure. For example, if a one-ounce bag of pretzels provides 100 calories and 10 of those calories are derived from fat, it contains 10 percent fat.

Nutrition Information on Food Labels

These nutrients are typically included on labels. Use the weight column for comparing similar foods, such as canned soups, and the "calories" column to see their proportion in each food group.

Calories Number of calories (energy) that are contained in the food.

Fat (g) Total amount of fat in grams. Select foods with less than 3g of fat per 100 calories. The total amount of saturated fat (in grams) is also shown. Select foods with less than 1g per 100 calories.

Cholesterol (mg) Total amount of cholesterol in milligrams. Try to select foods with less than 100mg per serving.

Carbohydrate (g) Total amount of carbohydrates from starches, sugars, and fiber. Choose foods that have a greater starch than sugar content.

Nutrition Information Typical Values	Amount per 100g	Percentage of calories
Calories (cal)	113	
Fat	1g	8
(of which saturated)	<1g	
Cholesterol	0 mg	
Sodium	0 mg	
Carbohydrate	23g	82
Dietary Fiber	1g	
Protein	3g	10

Sugar Where appropriate, information on sugar content may also be included on a food label.

Calories from fats The percentage of calories derived from fat. Nine calories are produced from every gram of fat. Select foods with fewer than 30% fat calories.

Sodium (g) Most sodium in food comes from salt (sodium chloride). If you have high blood pressure, it may be beneficial for you to choose foods with less than 500mg per serving.

Protein (g) There is usually more than enough protein in most people's diets. Be aware that foods that are high in protein may also have a high fat content.

Dietary Fiber (g) The total amount of fiber, including both soluble and insoluble types. Try to increase your total fiber intake to at least 24g per day.

CHOOSING HEALTHY OPTIONS

When shopping for ready-prepared foods or for the ingredients for your own cooking, always be on the lookout for healthy options – that is, foods or ingredients that are lower in fat than the traditional versions. You may find the following suggestions helpful.

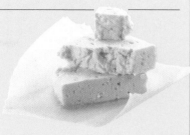

Meat, poultry, fish, and shellfish (<6–8 oz/day)	● Lean cuts of meat (with fat trimmed) Beef: round, sirloin, filet mignon; Lamb: leg, arm, loin, rib; Pork: loin, leg, lean ham; Veal: shoulder, leg ● Poultry: white meat chicken or turkey without skin ● Low fat or fat-free hot dogs ● Low fat or fat-free luncheon meats ● Fish: lean and fatty varieties ● Shellfish: lobster, scallops, clams, crabmeat, mussels, oysters, shrimp
Dairy products (3–4 servings/day)	● Fat-free or 1% milk, low-fat buttermilk ● Fat-free or low fat yogurt and cream cheese ● Low or reduced-fat cheeses (<5 grams fat per serving)
Eggs (<4 yolks per week)	● Egg whites ● Cholesterol-free egg substitutes
Fats and oils (6–8 tsp/day)	● Unsaturated vegetable oils ● Tub margarine (trans fat free) ● Fat-free, yogurt-based dressings, balsamic vinegar
Fruits and vegetables (>5 servings/day)	● Fresh, frozen, or dried varieties ● Oven-roasted vegetables, brushed with olive oil ● Low fat vegetable soups
Breads, cereals, whole grains, pastas, and rice	● Whole-grain bread or rolls, pita bread, breadsticks, rice cakes ● Bagels and English muffins ● Baked potatoes, rice, pasta ● Beans, peas, lentils ● Couscous, barley, millet
Sweets and desserts	● Fruit-based desserts, light or low fat yogurts, rice pudding made with fat-free or low fat milk ● Angel food cake with fresh or frozen fruit ● Low fat cookies, gingersnaps, or fig bars ● Non-fat or fat-free ice cream or frozen yogurt ● Fruit sorbets, sherbet, and Italian water ices

Source: National Heart, Lung and Blood Institute; NCEP Report

Low fat Cooking Techniques

THE FOLLOWING TECHNIQUES DEMONSTRATE SIMPLE WAYS TO KEEP FAT LEVELS TO A MINIMUM
WHEN COOKING WITHOUT COMPROMISING ON TASTE. THESE METHODS OF PREPARATION REDUCE
OR ELIMINATE THE NEED FOR ADDITIONAL OIL OR FAT AND ARE PREFERABLE TO FRYING AND
ROASTING, WHICH CAN INCREASE FAT LEVELS SIGNIFICANTLY.

WAYS OF REDUCING FAT IN COOKING

There are many quick and simple methods of food preparation that will ensure that fat levels are kept to a minimum when cooking.

○ Visible fat found on meat and the skin on poultry should be removed to reduce significantly the fat and calorie content.

○ Vegetables can be cooked in a little water instead of oil. The pan should be covered to enable the vegetables to cook in their own steam and moisture.

○ Flavorings such as herbs, garlic, wine, and lemon or lime juice can add flavor and moisture to fish, meat, or poultry, eliminating the need for additional oil.

○ A heavy-based, non-stick pan will help prevent foods from sticking, reducing the need for oil or fat.

○ Meat, poultry, or fish should be placed on a rack when broiling or roasting to allow fat from the foods to drain away.

PAN BROILING

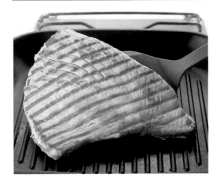

Pan broiling browns and seals in the juices of foods such as fish, meat, and poultry, and requires little or no extra oil or fat. It is important to preheat the skillet or griddle beforehand.

BROILING

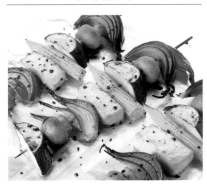

Broiling browns foods quickly on the outside while sealing the juices inside. It may be necessary to brush the foods with a little oil, or marinate them first, to prevent them from drying out.

SEARING

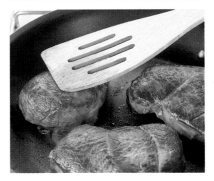

This method of cooking is perfect for sealing in the juices of foods such as meat, fish, and poultry, and requires little or no extra oil or fat. It is important to preheat the pan first.

STIR-FRYING

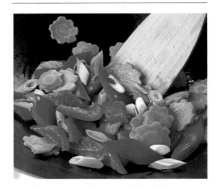

Stir-frying is a fast and healthy method of cooking, and a non-stick wok helps to keep fat levels to a minimum. It is important to prepare all ingredients before starting to cook.

HOT-SMOKING

Hot-smoking is a quick, totally fat-free method of cooking. Foods such as a fish, meat, and poultry are arranged on a rack placed in a wok, and cooked over a layer of tea leaves and other flavorings to give them a light, smoky flavor.

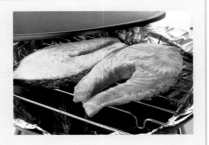

PARCEL-COOKING

Sometimes known as *en papillote*, this technique refers to foods cooked inside a parcel. This enables the flavor, juices, and nutrients to be retained and eliminates the need for additional oil or fat. It is suitable for foods such as fish, meat, poultry, and fruits and vegetables.

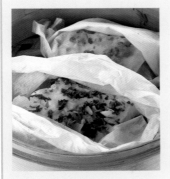

Cooking in parchment paper helps seal in the moisture in foods. The parcel can be placed in a steamer or baked in an oven. In the heat, the ingredients steam and the flavors mingle.

SAUTEING

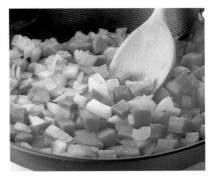

Foods that are cooked by sautéing should be moistened with a small amount of oil. A lid may also be used to allow the foods to cook in their own juices.

STEAMING

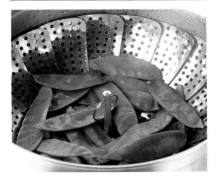

Steaming is a quick, fat-free method of cooking that is particularly suitable for vegetables, poultry, and fish. Careful timing is crucial to ensure that foods are cooked to perfection.

MARINATING

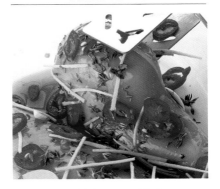

Marinades add flavor and help tenderize foods and keep them moist during cooking without the need for any or additional oil. Use them for poultry, meat, fish, and vegetables.

POACHING

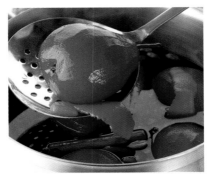

Poaching is a low fat method of cooking foods such as fruit, fish, eggs, and meat. Fruit is often poached in a syrup, while meat, poultry, and fish are usually simmered in stock.

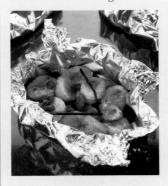

Cooking in foil works on the same principle as cooking in paper but foods may also be barbecued.

MEAL PLANNING

MEAL PLANNING IS ONE OF THE KEY FACTORS IN
MAINTAINING THE HEALTH OF THE HEART. BY
EATING A VARIED DIET BASED ON A RANGE OF
HEALTHY INGREDIENTS YOU CAN HELP CONTROL
YOUR WEIGHT, REDUCE CHOLESTEROL LEVELS,
AND RESTRICT YOUR TOTAL FAT INTAKE.

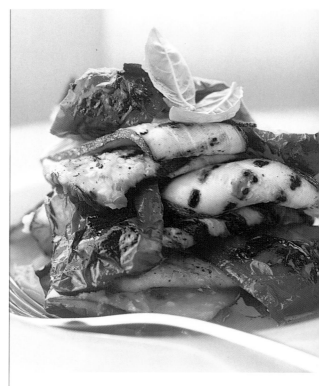

Healthy eating tips

The following guidelines will help you plan a well-balanced, healthy diet, even when eating out, and they complement the meal suggestions that follow.

● Cut down on the amount of fat you eat, especially your intake of saturated fat.

● Base meals and snacks around starchy foods, including bread, potatoes, rice, pasta, and cereals.

● Aim to eat at least five helpings of fruits and vegetables daily, including fresh, frozen, dried, and canned varieties, as well as fruit juices. Choose fruits canned in natural juice and avoid canned vegetables in salt or brine.

● Eat fish regularly – at least three servings a week. One or more of these servings should be oily fish: tuna, salmon, mackerel, herrings, or sardines.

● Choose low fat dairy produce such as skim milk, low fat yogurt, and low fat cheese.

● Eat only small amounts of lean meat and poultry.

● Reduce your salt intake.

● Choose foods that are a rich source of soluble fiber, such as oats, lentils, peas, corn, and beans.

VEGETARIAN SUPPERS

ARTICHOKE & FAVA BEAN STEW
(*page 84*), served with rice and steamed broccoli

BAKED BANANAS WITH VANILLA (*page 107*)

———

MEDITERRANEAN BROILED VEGETABLE
SALAD (*page 100*), served with bread,
rice, or pasta

PEACH & GINGER MERINGUE PIE
(*page 110*)

———

ORIENTAL MUSHROOM RISOTTO (*page 55*),
served with salad

FIGS WITH MARBLED YOGURT
& HONEY SAUCE (*page 106*)

ABOVE *Mediterranean Broiled Vegetable Salad*

BRUNCHES

FRUIT SMOOTHIE *(page 28)*

CRUSTLESS HERB & MUSHROOM QUICHE
(page 34) served with grilled tomatoes and
wholewheat toast

SPICED SMOKED FISH
(page 36) served with grilled tomatoes

STRAWBERRY & MANGO SALAD *(page 32)*

APRICOT & DATE MUESLI *(page 30)*

CARROT & BRAN MUFFINS
(page 35) served with grilled tomatoes

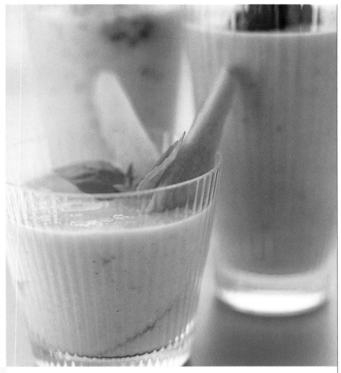

RIGHT *Fruit Smoothies*

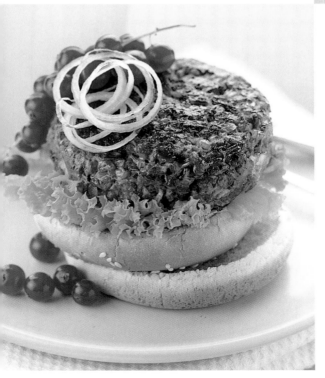

MIDWEEK DINNERS

BAKED COD WITH
TOMATO & PEPPER SALSA *(page 60)*
served with new potatoes and a green vegetable

CARAMELIZED RICE PUDDING *(page 115)*

ORIENTAL GINGER CHICKEN *(page 74)* served
with noodles and a green vegetable

POACHED SPICED PEARS *(page 107)*

VENISON BURGERS *(page 80)* served on a bun
with CARAMELIZED ONION & POTATO
SALAD *(page 91)*

MIXED MELON SALAD *(page 106)*

LEFT *Venison Burger*

Eating out

There is no reason to avoid eating out if you have a heart problem, but you should take care when ordering.

When eating out avoid foods that are high in fat, including: heavily dressed salads; creamy soups, sauces (hollandaise sauce and beurre blanc), and desserts; fried, batter-coated foods; fried vegetables; pastry; oily Italian breads, garlic bread, and bread spread thickly with butter; and the cheeseboard.

Instead choose dishes that are lower in fat:
- **APPETIZERS** Stock-based soups such as minestrone, chicken, or vegetable; salads with the dressing on the side; fruits such as melon, pineapple, or grapefruit; corn on the cob (without butter); or seafood (without heavy dressing) such as smoked salmon, crab, mussels, or oysters.

- **MAIN COURSES** Broiled poultry or fish with vegetables and potatoes, rice, or pasta; pasta with tomato sauce and salad; Chinese or Indian meal with boiled rice (avoid fried meat dishes and oily sauces); poultry kebabs; or tandoori chicken with rice.

- **DESSERTS** Fresh fruit salad; sorbet; meringue; low fat yogurt; or poached fruits.

Snack ideas

Many snacks are high in fat and contain very little in the way of nourishment. To avoid the temptation, choose from the following low fat, low salt alternatives.

- Toast with a little low fat spread and high-fruit jam

- A few plain cookies (about 1g fat per cookie)

- Fruits or low fat yogurts

- Crispbreads or rice cakes with low fat cheese

- Unsalted popcorn or pretzels

- Ice popsicles or sorbets

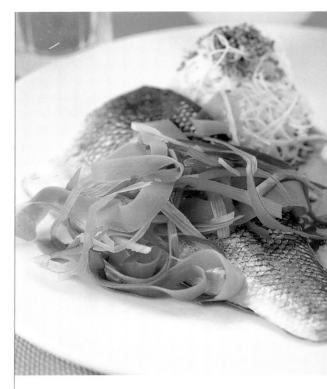

DINNER PARTIES

WINTER TOMATO SOUP (*page 40*)
served with wholegrain bread

CHINESE STEAMED SEA BASS (*page 68*)
served with a green vegetable and noodles

LAYERED FRUIT & YOGURT MOUSSE
(*page 105*)

CHILLED SUMMER CHERRY SOUP (*page 38*)
served with bread

FILET MIGNON WITH THREE-PEPPER
SALSA (*page 79*) served with
ROASTED GARLIC & ZUCCHINI SALAD
(*page 90*) and new potatoes

MIXED BERRIES WITH SWEET POLENTA
PIE (*page 112*)

ABOVE *Chinese Steamed Sea Bass*

LIGHT LUNCHES

THAI FISH & NOODLE SOUP *(page 44)*
served with a piece of fruit

MY FAVORITE SANDWICH *(page 48)*
served with salad

PEAR YOGURT ICE *(page 104)*

QUICK TOMATO & FRESH HERB PILAF
(page 51) followed by low fat plain yogurt
flavored with a spoonful of honey

COTTAGE CHEESE & FRESH HERBS
WITH PASTA *(page 58)* served with
a piece of fruit

BELOW *Thai Fish & Noodle Soup*

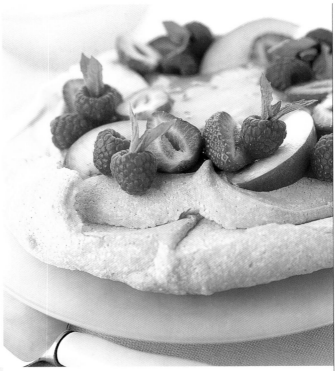

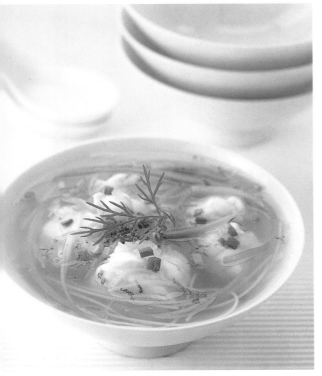

BUFFET PARTY FOR TEN

FRESH VEGETABLE PATTIES *(page 50)*

TANDOORI CHICKEN *(page 73)*

TEA-SMOKED SALMON *(page 71)*

ROASTED RED PEPPER & CHICKPEA
SALAD *(page 88)*

CARAMELIZED ONION & POTATO SALAD
(page 91)

BEET SALAD WITH HONEY & YOGURT
DRESSING *(page 93)*

TUNA & BEAN SALAD *(page 94)*

SMOKED EGGPLANT & TOMATO SALAD
(page 96)

PASSION FRUIT PAVLOVA *(page 108)*

CARAMELIZED PINEAPPLE *(page 114)*

ABOVE *Passion Fruit Pavlova*

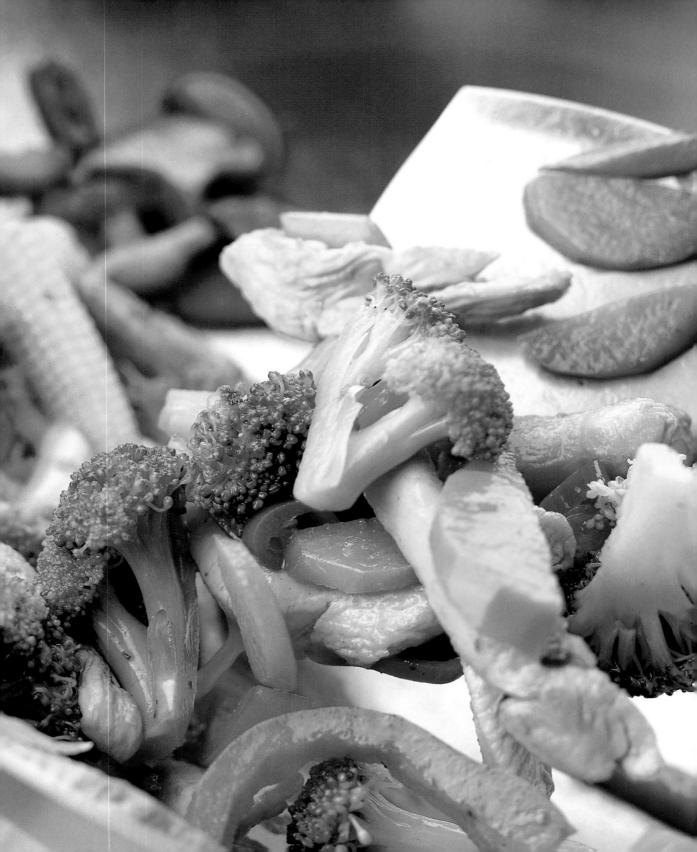

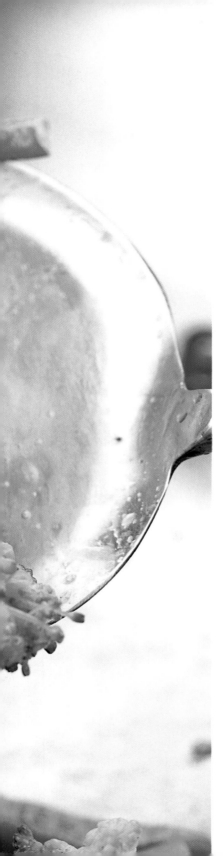

RECIPES

THE RECIPES IN THIS SECTION OFFER A NEW AND *fresh approach* TO HEALTHY EATING. THEY HAVE BEEN CREATED TO ENABLE YOU TO MAKE DELICIOUS, *inspiring,* AND *nutritious* BRUNCHES, SOUPS, LIGHT MEALS, MAIN COURSES, AND DESSERTS. THERE ARE ALSO *innovative ideas* FOR *low fat* SALAD DRESSINGS, SAUCES, AND STOCKS THAT WILL HELP YOU TO TRANSFORM ORDINARY DISHES INTO *gourmet meals.*

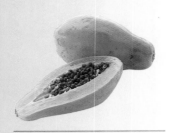

✱ STAR INGREDIENT
Papaya is a rich source of vitamin C and beta-carotene, both of which are antioxidants that may help to prevent cell damage and heart disease.

EACH SERVING PROVIDES:

○ Calories 160

○ Total Fat <1g
  Saturated Fat <1g
  Polyunsaturated Fat <1g
  Monounsaturated Fat <1g

○ Cholesterol 0mg

○ Sodium 44mg

○ Carbohydrate 35g
  Fiber 4g

○ Protein 7g

SERVING TIP
It is important to drink juices and smoothies soon after they are made since their nutritional value quickly diminishes.

Preparation Time: 10 minutes
Serves: 4

Papaya & Banana Smoothie

THIS VIBRANT AND REFRESHING DRINK MAKES A NUTRITIOUS AND INVIGORATING START TO THE DAY. TO FURTHER BOOST ITS FIBER CONTENT, ADD WHEATGERM OR ANOTHER SIMILAR GRAIN WHEN BLENDING THE FRUITS.

2 papayas, peeled, deseeded, and chilled
1 cup (200ml) fat-free plain yogurt, chilled
3 bananas
juice of 1 orange
1–2 tbsp honey (optional)
fresh basil or mint leaves, to decorate (optional)

Slice 1 papaya and reserve for garnish. Place all the remaining ingredients, with the exception of the basil leaves, in a blender, and process into a smooth purée. Serve decorated with the reserved slices of fresh papaya and the basil leaves.

VARIATIONS
Kiwi and Passion Fruit Smoothie Replace the papaya with 4 peeled kiwis and the pulp of 3 passion fruits. Blend the kiwis with the bananas, yogurt, orange juice, and honey, if using, until smooth, then stir in the passion fruit pulp. Decorate with a slice of fresh orange.

Raspberry and Pear Smoothie Replace the papaya and bananas with ½ cup (125g) raspberries or strawberries and 3 ripe pears, peeled and cored. Replace the orange juice with the juice of half a lemon. Blend these ingredients with the yogurt and honey, if using, and decorate with fresh raspberries and mint leaves.

BRUNCHES

Combining a late breakfast and an early lunch, brunches can recharge the body and provide nutrients and long-term, sustained energy. These recipes include quick ideas for every day, and suggestions for more leisurely occasions.

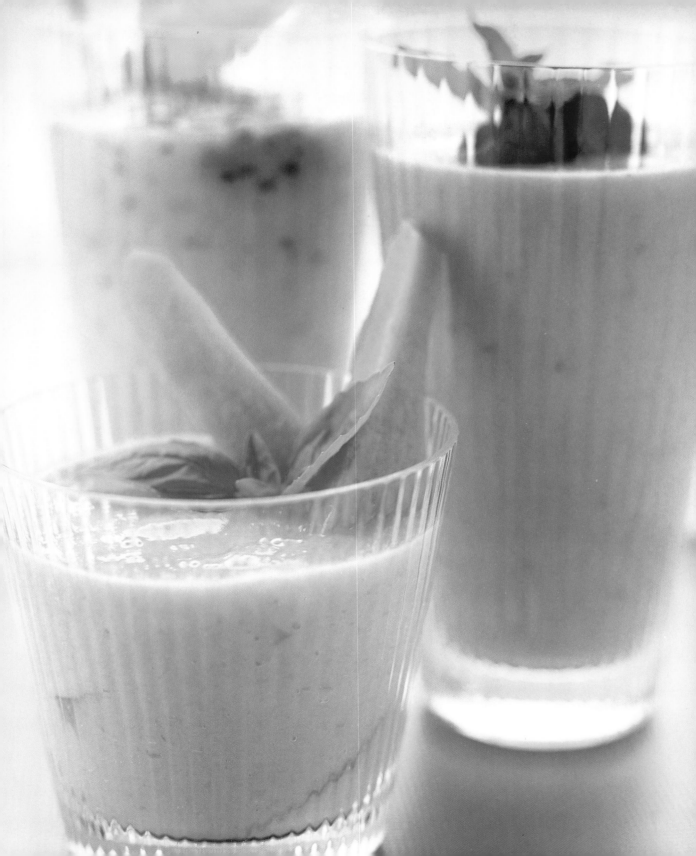

EACH SERVING PROVIDES:

○ Calories 100

○ Total Fat <1g
Saturated Fat <0.5g
Polyunsaturated Fat <1g
Monounsaturated Fat <1g

○ Cholesterol 0mg

○ Sodium 24mg

○ Carbohydrate 24g
Fiber 1g

○ Protein 1g

Preparation Time: 5 minutes,
plus chilling overnight
Serves: 4

EXOTIC DRIED FRUIT SALAD

THIS DELICIOUS, HIGH-FIBER FRUIT SALAD SHOULD BE MADE THE
NIGHT BEFORE IT IS EATEN. SERVE IT WITH A SPOONFUL OF
LOW-FAT PLAIN YOGURT AND SLICES OF WHOLEWHEAT BREAD.
A SPRINKLING OF GRANOLA ADDS A PLEASANT CRUNCH.

¼ cup (30g) dried pineapple, sliced into bite-sized pieces
¼ cup (30g) dried mango, sliced into bite-sized pieces
¼ cup (30g) dried, pitted cherries or cranberries
¼ cup (30g) dried prunes
1½ cups (350ml) unsweetened pineapple juice
juice of ½ lemon and ½ tsp grated peel
1–2 tbsp honey or sugar (optional)

1 Put the dried fruit in a large, ceramic or glass bowl.

2 Put the pineapple juice, lemon juice and grated peel, and honey,
if using in a small saucepan, and heat gently but do not boil. Pour the
liquid over the fruit. Let the fruit cool, covered, and refrigerate overnight.

EACH SERVING PROVIDES:

○ Calories 190

○ Total Fat 2g
Saturated Fat <1g
Polyunsaturated Fat 1g
Monounsaturated Fat <1g

○ Cholesterol 0mg

○ Sodium 20mg

○ Carbohydrate 40g
Fiber 5g

○ Protein 6g

Preparation Time: 5 minutes
Serves: 15

APRICOT & DATE MUESLI

THIS IS A BALANCED AND ENERGY-PACKED MIXTURE OF DRIED FRUIT
AND HIGH-FIBER CEREALS. MAKE A LARGE QUANTITY OF THIS
MUESLI AND STORE IT IN AN AIRTIGHT CONTAINER.

¾ cup (150g) jumbo oats
1½ cups (150g) barley flakes
¼ cup (150g) oat bran
1½ cups (150g) wheat flakes
⅔ cup (100g) raisins
½ cup (100g) dried apricots, chopped
½ cup (100g) dried dates, chopped

Mix the cereals and dried fruit together in a large bowl, then store in an
airtight container for up to 2 weeks.

JUMBO OATS WITH SUMMER FRUIT

ROLLED OATS HAVE AN IMPORTANT ROLE TO PLAY IN A HEALTHY

HEART DIET BECAUSE THEY ARE REPUTED TO LOWER CHOLESTEROL

LEVELS. SPRINKLED WITH OAT FLAKES, COOKED CEREAL ALSO

MAKES A WARMING WINTER BREAKFAST.

3 cups (750ml) skim milk or water
6 tbsp jumbo oats
¾–1 cup (150g) berries, such as
raspberries, strawberries, or blueberries

1 Bring the milk to a boil. Sprinkle the oats over the milk, and stir well. Reduce the heat and simmer, stirring frequently, for 20–25 minutes, until thick and creamy.

2 Add the berries, reserving a few to decorate, and cook for a further minute. Decorate with the reserved berries.

EACH SERVING PROVIDES:

- Calories 160
- Total Fat 3g
  Saturated Fat 1g
  Polyunsaturated Fat 1g
  Monounsaturated Fat 1g
- Cholesterol 8mg
- Sodium 112mg
- Carbohydrate 30g
  Fiber 3g
- Protein 10g

Preparation Time: 30 minutes
Serves: 4

MALTED MILLET CEREAL

MILLET IS ONE OF NATURE'S MOST NUTRITIONALLY BALANCED FOODS:

ABUNDANT IN VITAMINS AND MINERALS, IT IS ALSO HIGH IN FIBER.

THIS HOT CEREAL MAKES AN IDEAL START TO THE DAY.

2 cups (500ml) skim milk or water
2 tbsp malt extract
6 tbsp millet flour
2–3 tbsp honey (optional)

1 In a small saucepan, bring the milk to a boil. Add the malt extract and stir well until melted. Sprinkle with the millet flour and stir.

2 Reduce the heat and simmer, stirring frequently, for 20–25 minutes, until thick and creamy. Serve drizzled with honey, if desired.

EACH SERVING PROVIDES:

- Calories 140
- Total Fat 1g
  Saturated Fat <1g
  Polyunsaturated Fat <1g
  Monounsaturated Fat <1g
- Cholesterol 5mg
- Sodium 73mg
- Carbohydrate 30g
  Fiber 1g
- Protein 6g

PREPARATION TIPS
Ground millet can be found in health food stores. Coarse corn meal can also be used.

Preparation Time: 30 minutes
Serves: 4

EACH SERVING PROVIDES:

○ Calories 60

○ Total Fat <0.5g
  Saturated Fat 0g
  Polyunsaturated Fat 0g
  Monounsaturated Fat 0g

○ Cholesterol 0mg

○ Sodium 5mg

○ Carbohydrate 15g
  Fiber 2g

○ Protein 1g

Preparation Time: 5 minutes
Serves: 4

STRAWBERRY & MANGO SALAD

A WONDERFULLY REFRESHING, SWEET, AND VIBRANT SUMMER BREAKFAST DISH THAT IS EQUALLY DELICIOUS MADE WITH OTHER COMBINATIONS OF FRESH, SEASONAL FRUIT. SERVE IT WITH A DOLLOP OF LOW-FAT PLAIN YOGURT AND SLICES OF WHOLEWHEAT TOAST.

juice of 1 orange
juice of ½ lemon
honey or sugar, to taste (optional)
1 large mango, peeled, pitted, and cubed
1 cup (250g) strawberries, hulled and quartered

Place the orange juice, lemon juice, and honey, if using, in a bowl. Add the mango and strawberries as they are prepared, and fold them into the citrus liquid. Serve immediately.

EACH SERVING PROVIDES:

○ Calories 110

○ Total Fat 4g
  Saturated Fat 0g
  Polyunsaturated Fat 1g
  Monounsaturated Fat 3g

○ Cholesterol 0mg

○ Sodium 162mg

○ Carbohydrate 0g
  Fiber 2g

○ Protein 1g

Preparation Time: 15 minutes,
plus 2 hours marinating
Serves: 4

BROILED SPICED PINEAPPLE

1 tbsp reduced-salt soy sauce
1 tbsp molasses or soft, dark-brown sugar
½ tsp ground star anise
juice of ½ lemon
1 pineapple, peeled, cored, and sliced into
1in (2.5cm) rings
1 tbsp grapeseed or sunflower oil

1 In a large bowl, mix together the soy sauce, molasses, star anise, and lemon juice. Add the pineapple and carefully turn the rings in the marinade until coated. Let it marinate for at least 2 hours.

2 Preheat the broiler to high, brush the pineapple with the oil, and broil for 3–4 minutes on each side. Serve immediately.

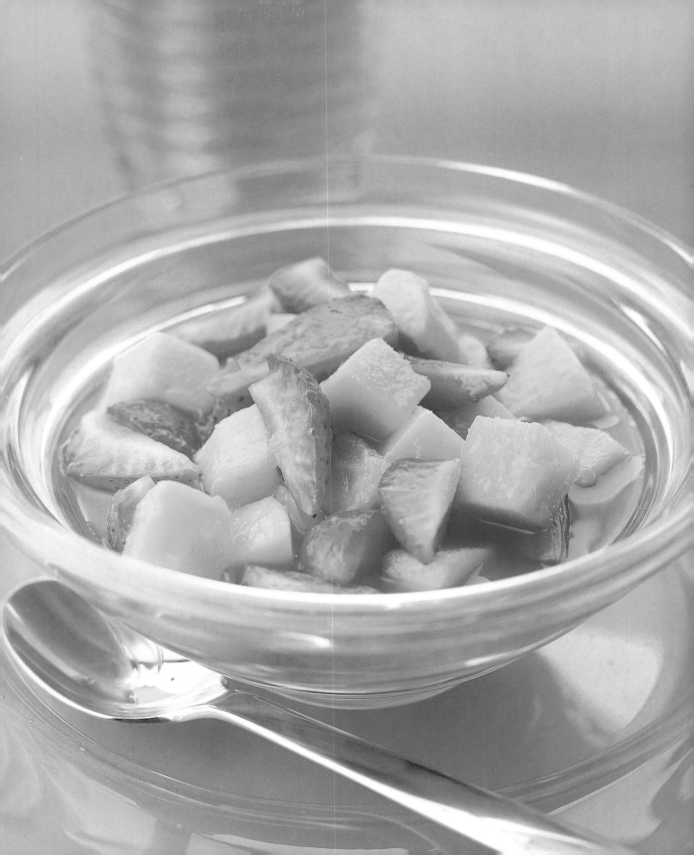

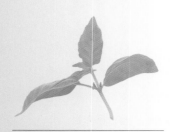

✶ STAR INGREDIENT
Use basil regularly in cooking to boost intake of the antioxidants vitamin C and beta-carotene. Basil is a tonic and is also calming to the nervous system.

EACH SERVING PROVIDES:

○ Calories 92

○ Total Fat 0.5g

○ Cholesterol mg

○ Sodium 279mg

○ Carbohydrate 9g
   Fiber 1g

○ Protein 12g

Preparation Time: 1 hour, 10 minutes
Serves: 8

CRUSTLESS HERB & MUSHROOM QUICHE

HERBS ADD FLAVOR AND A BRIGHT COLOR TO THIS

LOW FAT VERSION OF QUICHE, WHICH AVOIDS THE NEED

FOR A HIGH FAT PASTRY CASE.

1 cup (70g) mushrooms, sliced
16oz (450ml) fat-free egg substitute
⅓ cup (45g) all-purpose flour
1 tsp baking powder
16oz (450g) non-fat cottage cheese
2 tbsp chopped fresh basil
½ cup (10g) chopped fresh parsley
¼ cup (20g) scallions, thinly sliced
¼ tsp cayenne pepper
¼ tsp salt

1 Preheat the oven to 400°F (200°C). Lightly spray a 10 inch (25cm) pie pan with cooking spray.

2 Cook the mushrooms for 2–3 minutes in a non-stick skillet to eliminate some of their moisture.

3 Combine the mushrooms with the remaining ingredients, then pour this mixture into the pie pan.

4 Bake for 15 minutes, then lower the oven temperature to 350°F (180°C) and bake for 35–40 minutes longer, until a toothpick inserted into the center comes out clean. Let cool for 10 minutes on a rack before serving.

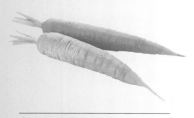

CARROT & BRAN MUFFINS

THESE MUFFINS ARE FULL OF FLAVOR, MOIST, AND DELICIOUS –

SO MUCH SO THAT THE FACT THAT THEY ARE LOW IN FAT AND

HIGH IN VITAMINS DOES NOT SEEM EVIDENT.

1 cup (85g) bran flake cereal, crushed
¾ cup (75g) wholewheat flour
¾ cup (90g) all-purpose flour
½ tsp cinnamon
½ tsp soda
1 tsp baking powder
3 tbsp brown sugar
¼ tsp salt
2 egg whites, lightly beaten
2 tbsp vegetable oil
⅓ cup (80ml) buttermilk
1 cup apple sauce
1 tbsp lemon juice
1 cup (150g) carrots, grated
½ cup (50g) raisins

1 Preheat the oven to 375°F (190°C). Spray a twelve cup muffin pan with oil spray.

2 Combine the bran flakes with the wholewheat and all-purpose flours, cinnamon, soda, baking powder, sugar, and salt.

3 In a separate bowl, blend together the egg whites, oil, buttermilk, apple sauce, and lemon juice. Combine this mixture with the dry ingredients. Stir in the carrots and raisins, until combined.

4 Pour the mixture into the muffin cups. Bake for 20 minutes, until risen and golden.

✶ STAR INGREDIENT
Carrots are probably the best-known source of beta-carotene, the antioxidant that fights free radicals, thus preventing cell damage.

EACH MUFFIN PROVIDES:

○ Calories 125

○ Total Fat 2.5g

○ Cholesterol mg

○ Sodium 210mg

○ Carbohydrate 27g
   Fiber 1g

○ Protein 3g

Preparation Time: 30 minutes
Makes: 12

White fish, such as haddock, is
an excellent source of low fat
protein, and also provides
selenium, iodine, and vitamin E.

EACH SERVING PROVIDES:

○ Calories 270

○ Total Fat 1g
  Saturated Fat <1g
  Polyunsaturated Fat <1g
  Monounsaturated Fat <1g

○ Cholesterol 32mg

○ Sodium 65mg

○ Carbohydrate 43g
  Fiber 1g

○ Protein 21g

PREPARATION TIP
For a vegetarian version, use
¾lb (350g) smoked or plain
tofu, cubed, instead of the fish.
Add it to the cooked rice in
step 3.

Preparation Time: 50 minutes,
plus 30 minutes marinating
Serves: 4

SPICED SMOKED FISH

BECAUSE SMOKED FISH IS HIGH IN SALT, THIS ALTERNATIVE IS

MADE WITH FRESH HADDOCK, WHILE THE STAR ANISE

LENDS A DELICIOUS SMOKY FLAVOR TO THE DISH. SERVE

IT WITH BROILED TOMATOES.

juice of 1 lemon
1 tsp mild curry powder
1 tsp ground star anise
½ tsp ground turmeric
11½oz (350g) haddock fillets
3 cups (750ml) water
1 small lemon, sliced into thin rounds
1 bay leaf
10 peppercorns
1 large onion, finely chopped
200g (7oz) long-grain rice
3 tbsp chopped fresh parsley, plus sprigs to garnish
salt and freshly ground black pepper, to taste
lemon wedges, to serve

1 Combine the lemon juice, curry powder, star anise, and turmeric,
then spoon the mixture over the haddock. Turn the fish in the marinade
to coat both sides. Cover, and refrigerate for at least 30 minutes.

2 Place the water, lemon slices, bay leaf, and peppercorns in a large
frying pan and bring to a boil. Reduce the heat, and simmer for
10 minutes. Add the fish and marinade, then cook for 8–10 minutes
more, until the fish is tender. Lift out the fish, remove any skin and
bones, then flake the flesh. Strain and reserve the liquid.

3 Place the onion in a saucepan with 5 tablespoons of the reserved
liquid. Bring to a boil, cover, then simmer for 6 minutes. Add the rice,
parsley, and the remaining cooking liquid. Bring to a boil, then reduce
the heat and simmer, covered, for 20 minutes, until the rice is tender.
Add the fish and chopped parsley, and heat through. Season, garnish
with parsley sprigs, and serve with the lemon wedges.

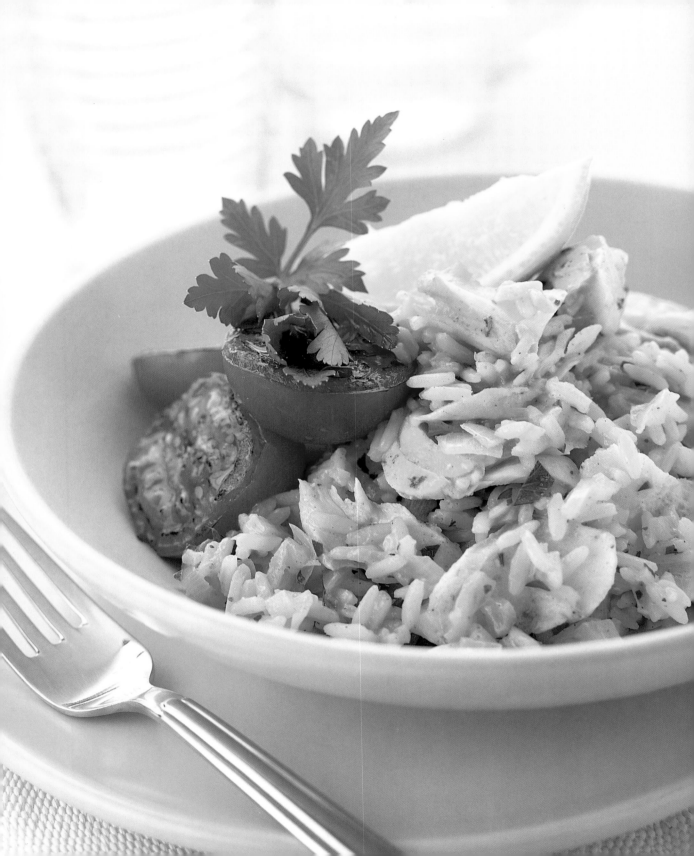

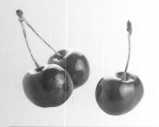

★ STAR INGREDIENT
Cherries provide valuable amounts of vitamin C.

EACH SERVING PROVIDES:

○ Calories 90

○ Total Fat <1g
Saturated Fat 0g
Polyunsaturated Fat <1g
Monounsaturated Fat <1g

○ Cholesterol 0mg

○ Sodium 126mg

○ Carbohydrate 20g
Fiber 1g

○ Protein 2g

PREPARATION TIP
Avoid buying stock cubes that are high in salt. Homemade stocks or good-quality store-bought ones are preferable.

Preparation Time: 25 minutes, plus 1 hour chilling
Serves: 4

CHILLED SUMMER CHERRY SOUP

WHAT COULD BE BETTER ON A HOT SUMMER DAY THAN THIS CHILLED FRUIT SOUP? CHERRIES ARE REPUTED TO PROMOTE GENERAL GOOD HEALTH. SERVE THE SOUP WITH SLICES OF LIGHTLY TOASTED BREAD.

2⅔ cups (500g) cherries, pitted and coarsely chopped
2¼ cups (500ml) chicken or vegetable stock
(see pages 118–19), or water
2 tbsp honey or sugar
½ cinnamon stick
2 tsp cornstarch
2 tbsp lemon juice
peel of 1 lemon, cut into fine strips,
plus extra, to garnish (optional)
4 tbsp fat-free fromage frais or plain yogurt

1 Place the cherries in a large, stainless steel or enamel saucepan. Add the stock, honey, and cinnamon. Bring to a boil, then reduce the heat and simmer for 15 minutes, or until the cherries have softened.

2 Mix the cornstarch with the lemon juice, and stir into the soup. Simmer for a few more minutes until slightly thickened. Add the lemon peel, and remove from the heat. Leave to cool, then chill for 1 hour. Divide the soup between 4 bowls and place a tablespoon of fromage frais on top of each portion. Garnish with strips of lemon peel, if using, before serving.

SOUPS *Nutritious, sustaining, and incredibly versatile, homemade soups are the perfect food for a healthy heart and body. Served with a chunk of wholewheat bread and a fresh green or mixed salad, a soup makes a light yet satisfying low fat meal.*

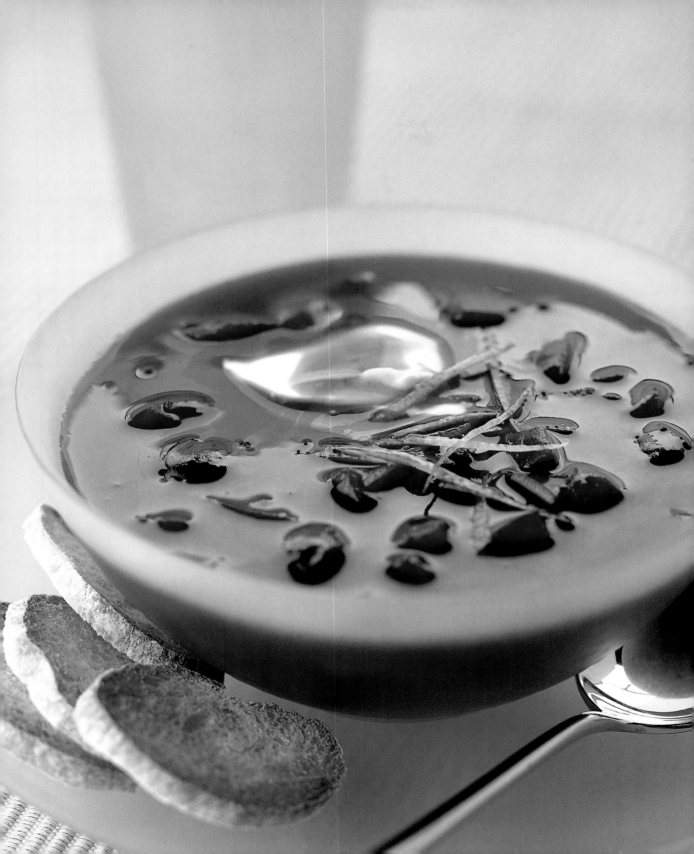

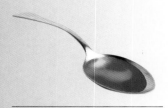

WINTER TOMATO SOUP

TRY THIS LOW FAT VERSION OF AN OLD FAVORITE. IT IS CREAMY,

SWEET AND SOUR, AND VERY TASTY. IT IS ALSO PACKED WITH

LOTS OF VITAMINS AND MINERALS. SERVE THIS SOUP WITH

A CHUNK OF WHOLEGRAIN BREAD.

1 onion, finely chopped
3 cloves garlic, finely chopped
2 celery sticks, finely chopped
juice and grated peel of 1 orange
1 tbsp olive oil
2 cups (500g) tomatoes, skinned, deseeded,
and finely chopped
1½ cups (350ml) fresh orange juice
2¼ cups (500ml) chicken or vegetable stock
(see pages 118–19)
2 tbsp rice
freshly grated nutmeg, to taste
2–3 tbsp lemon juice, to taste
freshly ground black pepper, to taste
chopped fresh basil, to garnish

1 Place the onion, garlic, celery, orange juice, and grated peel in a large saucepan. Cook over a medium heat for 5 minutes, or until the orange juice has evaporated. Stir in the oil and cook for a further 4–5 minutes, until the onion has softened and started to brown.

2 Add 1½ cups (400g) of the tomatoes, the fresh orange juice, stock, and rice. Bring to a boil, then reduce the heat, and simmer for about 35–40 minutes, until the soup has reduced and thickened. Add the nutmeg, lemon juice, and the remaining tomatoes, and heat through. Season, and garnish with the basil leaves before serving.

VARIATION

Summer Tomato Soup Omit the rice, and cook the liquid as in step 2, above, for 25 minutes. Stir in the nutmeg, lemon juice, and the remaining tomatoes and heat through. Season and leave to cool, then refrigerate for at least 2 hours.

✳ STAR INGREDIENT
Olive oil is rich in monounsaturated fat, which is good for maintaining levels of good cholesterol in the body.

EACH SERVING PROVIDES:

○ Calories 140

○ Total Fat 4g
  Saturated Fat <1g
  Polyunsaturated Fat <1g
  Monounsaturated Fat 3g

○ Cholesterol 0mg

○ Sodium 130mg

○ Carbohydrate 23g
  Fiber 2g

○ Protein 3g

BUYING TIP
Whenever possible use fresh tomatoes such as Italian plum or beef varieties. Salad tomatoes tend to be too watery and lack the intensity of flavor needed for cooking.

Preparation Time: 60 minutes
Serves: 4

MUSHROOM & BARLEY SOUP

ALTHOUGH BARLEY IS PROBABLY THE MOST ANCIENT CULTIVATED

CEREAL CROP, IT IS NOT VERY COMMON. YET THIS NUTRITIOUS GRAIN

IS REPUTED TO LOWER BLOOD-CHOLESTEROL LEVELS, AND MAKES

A WONDERFULLY HEARTY, SATISFYING SOUP.

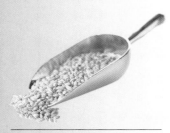

✱ STAR INGREDIENT
A regular intake of high-fiber grains, such as barley, is linked with a reduced risk of heart disease, high blood pressure, and certain cancers.

EACH SERVING PROVIDES:

○ Calories 120

○ Total Fat 4g
  Saturated Fat <1g
  Polyunsaturated Fat <1g
  Monounsaturated Fat 3g

○ Cholesterol 0mg

○ Sodium 198mg

○ Carbohydrate 20g
  Fiber 1g

○ Protein 2g

PREPARATION TIP
Soak the barley for 2 hours in cold water before use to reduce the cooking time by half.

Preparation Time: 1 hour, 15 minutes
Serves: 4

1 tbsp olive oil
1 onion, chopped, or the white part
of 2 leeks, finely chopped
2oz (60g) pearl barley, soaked in cold water
for 2 hours, and drained
3 cups (1 liter) vegetable stock (see page 118),
skim milk, or water
2 tbsp (20g) dried porcini mushrooms, soaked
for 30 minutes in ¼ cup hot water
1 bay leaf
1 large carrot, coarsely grated
freshly ground black pepper, to taste

1 Heat the oil in a heavy-based saucepan, then add the onions. Cover, and cook for 5 minutes, or until the onions have softened.

2 Add the barley and cook for another 1–2 minutes, until the barley is coated in the onion mixture. Add the stock, rehydrated mushrooms, with their strained liquid, and bay leaf. Bring to a boil, then reduce the heat and simmer for 50–55 minutes, or until the barley is tender.

3 Add the grated carrots, and continue to simmer the soup for 5–6 minutes, until the carrots are tender. Season before serving.

VARIATION
Smoked Mushroom and Barley Soup Add 1½oz (50g) smoked ham, cut into cubes with fat removed, with the carrot in step 3, above. (To remove the excess salt in the ham, blanch it first for 5 minutes in boiling water, then drain and rinse.)

MEDITERRANEAN BEAN SOUP

THIS FILLING SOUP IS PACKED WITH A NUTRITIOUS COMBINATION OF

VEGETABLES, GRAINS, AND BEANS. SERVE IT WITH ITALIAN-STYLE

BREADCRUMBS. CANNELLINI BEANS CAN BE USED

INSTEAD OF THE LIMA BEANS.

1 tbsp olive oil
1 large onion, chopped
3 cloves garlic, finely chopped
2 celery sticks, finely chopped
1 large carrot, finely chopped
4½ cups (1 liter) chicken or vegetable stock
(see pages 118–19)
2 tbsp pearl barley, soaked in cold water
for 2 hours, and drained
2–3 (150g) plum tomatoes, skinned,
seeded, and chopped
1½ cups (200g) canned lima beans in water
small bunch of fresh parsley,
coarsely chopped
freshly ground black pepper, to taste

1 Heat the oil in a large saucepan. Add the onion, garlic, celery, and carrot, then sauté over a medium heat for 5–8 minutes, until the onion has softened and browned. If the mixture becomes too dry, add 1–2 tablespoons of water.

2 Add the stock and barley. Bring to a boil, then reduce the heat, cover, and simmer for 50–55 minutes, until the barley is tender. Add the tomatoes, beans, and parsley, reserving a little of the herb for garnish. Simmer for another 5 minutes, or until heated through. Season, and serve garnished with the reserved parsley.

★ STAR INGREDIENT

Beans provide significant amounts of soluble fiber, which can substantially reduce cholesterol levels if eaten on a regular basis. They are also high in iron, folate, and potassium.

EACH SERVING PROVIDES:

○ Calories 210

○ Total Fat 5g
  Saturated Fat 1g
  Polyunsaturated Fat 1g
  Monounsaturated Fat 3g

○ Cholesterol 0mg

○ Sodium 264mg

○ Carbohydrate 27g
  Fiber 6g

○ Protein 16g

PREPARATION TIP

If using dried lima beans, soak ⅔ cup (100g) beans in cold water overnight, then drain and rinse. Cover with cold water in a saucepan and bring to a boil. Cover, reduce the heat, and simmer for 1–1½ hours, until tender. Add to the soup in step 2, with the tomatoes.

Preparation Time: 1 hour, 20 minutes
Serves: 4

LENTIL & CILANTRO SOUP

THIS CREAMY, LEMONY, HEARTY SOUP FORMS A MEAL IN ITSELF
WHEN ACCOMPANIED BY A SALAD AND BREAD. LENTILS ARE
ESPECIALLY GOOD FOR THE HEART BECAUSE THEY PROVIDE
SOLUBLE FIBER, VITAMINS, AND MINERALS.

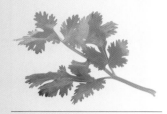

✴ STAR INGREDIENT

Fresh herbs such as cilantro are
an often overlooked source of
vitamin C.

EACH SERVING PROVIDES:

○ Calories 230

○ Total Fat 5g
   Saturated Fat 1g
   Polyunsaturated Fat 1g
   Monounsaturated Fat 3g

○ Cholesterol 0mg

○ Sodium 250mg

○ Carbohydrate 29g
   Fiber 3g

○ Protein 19g

PREPARATION TIP

Green or brown lentils can
be used instead of the
red lentils.

Preparation Time: 50 minutes
Serves: 4

1 tbsp olive oil
1 onion, finely chopped
3 cloves garlic, finely chopped
1 large carrot, grated
small bunch of fresh cilantro, chopped
½ cup (125g) red lentils, rinsed
2 tbsp bulgar, rinsed
4 ½ cups (1 liter) chicken or vegetable stock
(see pages 118–19)
juice and grated peel of 1 lemon
freshly ground black pepper, to taste

1 Heat the oil in a large saucepan. Add the onion, garlic, carrot, and
cilantro, reserving a little of the herb to garnish. Sauté over a medium
heat for 5–8 minutes, until the onion has softened and browned. If the
mixture becomes too dry, add 1–2 tablespoons of water.

2 Add the lentils and bulgar, stir well, then add the stock. Bring to
a boil, then reduce the heat, and simmer for 30 minutes, or until the
lentils are tender. Stir in the lemon juice and grated peel, then season.
Serve garnished with the reserved cilantro.

VARIATIONS

Smoked Lentril and Cilantro Soup Stir in 8oz (250g) smoked tofu,
cubed, about 10 minutes before the end of the specified cooking time.

Spicy Lentril and Cilantro Soup For a spicy version, add 1–2 red
chilies, deseeded and chopped, with the onion in step 1, above. Stir in
¼ teaspoon ground cumin with the lemon juice in step 2, above.

THAI FISH & NOODLE SOUP

THIS THAI-INSPIRED FISH SOUP IS SIMPLE TO MAKE, AND WHEN SERVED

WITH BREAD AND SALAD IT MAKES A DELICIOUS, LOW FAT MEAL.

MONKFISH IS USED IN THIS VERSION, BUT OTHER FIRM, LEAN FISH,

SUCH AS HALIBUT OR SWORDFISH, ARE EQUALLY SUITABLE.

★ STAR INGREDIENT
Fresh fish is not only low in fat, but also provides high levels of protein in a healthy form.

EACH SERVING PROVIDES:

○ Calories 150

○ Total Fat 4g
Saturated Fat <1g
Polyunsaturated Fat 3g
Monounsaturated Fat <1g

○ Cholesterol 14mg

○ Sodium 198mg

○ Carbohydrate 10g
Fiber 1g

○ Protein 17g

PREPARATION TIP
To add a slightly smoky flavor to the monkfish, after marinating it, cook it for a few minutes on a hot, lightly greased griddle, until golden. Add the fish to the soup in step 4.

Preparation Time: 40 minutes, plus 30 minutes marinating
Serves: 4

13oz (400g) monkfish fillet, cut into bite-sized cubes
juice of 1 lime, and 1 tsp grated peel
7 large (100g) shallots, finely chopped
2 cloves garlic, finely chopped
1 carrot, finely shredded
1in (2.5cm) piece of fresh ginger, finely chopped
2 sticks of lemongrass, outer leaves discarded,
and inside finely chopped
1 small red chili, seeded and finely chopped
4 tbsp water
1 tbsp grapeseed oil
3¼ cups (750ml) fish stock (see page 118)
¼ cup (30g) rice noodles, broken into short lengths,
and soaked for 3 minutes in boiling water
fresh dill or cilantro, to garnish

1 Place the monkfish in a dish. Spoon over the lime juice and half the grated peel. Cover, and leave to marinate in the refrigerator for 30 minutes.

2 Place the shallots, garlic, carrot, ginger, lemongrass, and chili in a large saucepan. Add the water, and bring to a boil. Reduce the heat, cover, and simmer, stirring occasionally, for 5 minutes, or until the water has evaporated. Add the oil and sauté, stirring, until the vegetables have softened.

3 Add the stock, and return to a boil. Reduce the heat, skim away any froth, and simmer for about 20 minutes.

4 Add the fish and noodles to the soup, then simmer for 5–8 minutes, until the fish is tender. Stir in the lime juice and grated peel marinade. Garnish with the dill and reserved grated peel before serving.

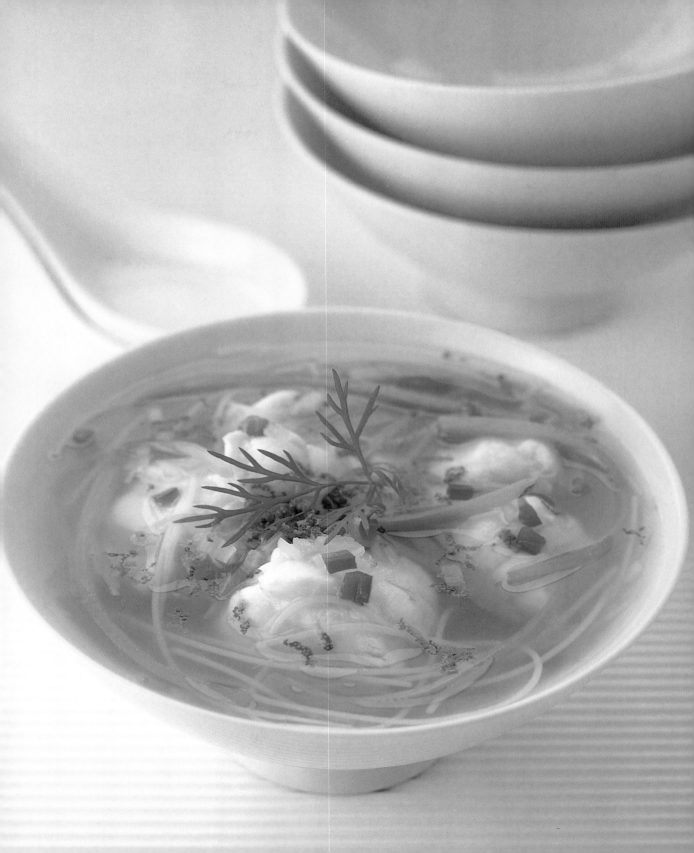

Roasted Vegetables with Herbs & Garlic

ROASTING ENHANCES THE FLAVOR OF FRESH VEGETABLES, MAKING

THEM SWEET AND AROMATIC. THIS DISH IS DELICIOUS SERVED

SIMPLY WITH PASTA OR BREAD AND A GREEN LEAF SALAD.

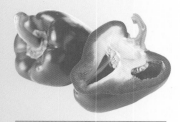

✱ STAR INGREDIENT
Red peppers are a good source of beta-carotene and vitamin C, both of which are antioxidants.

EACH SERVING PROVIDES:

○ Calories 120

○ Total Fat 8g
 Saturated Fat 1g
 Polyunsaturated Fat 1g
 Monounsaturated Fat 6g

○ Cholesterol 0mg

○ Sodium 15mg

○ Carbohydrate 9g
 Fiber 2g

○ Protein 3g

SERVING TIPS
This dish is delicious cold and will keep in the refrigerator for up to 2 days. Serve it as an accompaniment to meat or fish.

Preparation Time: 55 minutes
Serves: 4

4 tbsp water or fresh orange juice
⅔ cup (100g) yellow squash or green zucchini, grated
1 red pepper, cored, seeded, and sliced into ribbons
1½ cups (100g) broccoli florets
5 shallots, quartered
3–4 cloves garlic, quartered
1¼ cups (300g) vine cherry tomatoes
2 tbsp olive oil
2 tsp brown sugar
2 sprigs each of fresh rosemary and thyme
freshly ground black pepper, to taste
fresh basil leaves, to garnish

1 Preheat the oven to 400°F (200°C). Pour the water over the squash, pepper, broccoli, shallots, and garlic in a baking tray. Cover with foil, and bake for 25 minutes.

2 Increase the heat to 450°F (230°C). Remove the foil from the vegetables, then add the tomatoes, oil, sugar, herbs, and seasoning. Bake, turning the vegetables frequently, for 20–25 minutes, or until they have browned and caramelized. Garnish with the basil before serving.

LIGHT MEALS

This eclectic range of dishes does not rely on excessive amounts of meat and fish to give substance, but is based on healthy and delicious vegetables, beans, and starchy carbohydrates, including bread, rice, bulgar, and pasta.

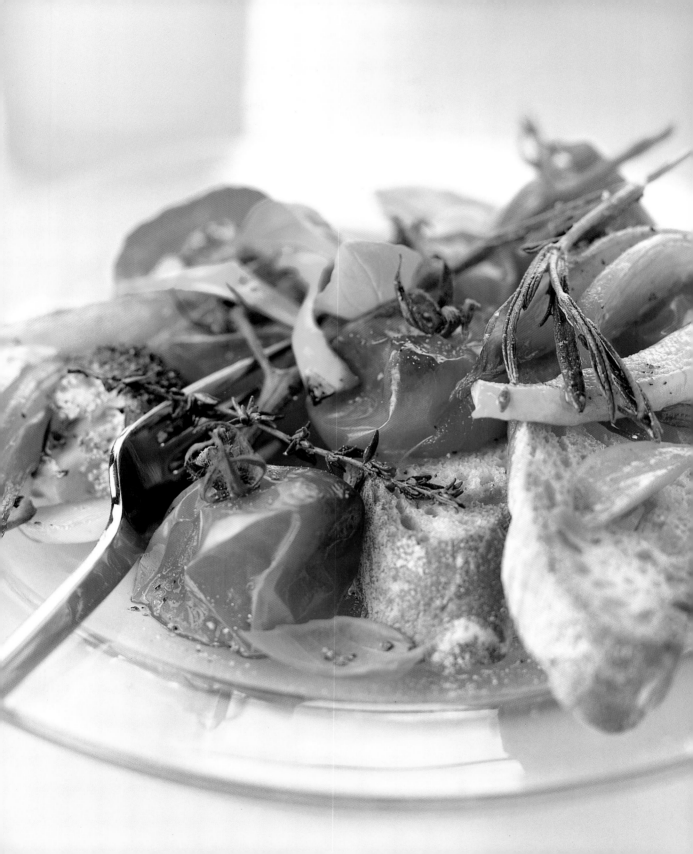

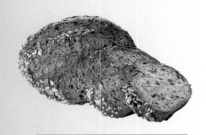

★ STAR INGREDIENT
A good-quality wholegrain bread
will boost your fiber intake and
prevent constipation.

EACH SERVING PROVIDES:

○ Calories 270

○ Total Fat 7g
    Saturated Fat 1g
    Polyunsaturated Fat 2g
    Monounsaturated Fat 4g

○ Cholesterol 0mg

○ Sodium 455mg

○ Carbohydrate 44g
    Fiber 2g

○ Protein 9g

PREPARATION TIP
This sandwich improves in
flavor if made an hour before
serving. Wrap in plastic wrap
and refrigerate.

Preparation Time: 10 minutes
Serves: 1

My Favorite Sandwich

THIS SANDWICH FEATURES A HEALTHY COMBINATION OF TOMATOES,

ONIONS, AND PARSLEY, WHICH ARE ALL BELIEVED TO BENEFIT THE

HEART. ADD A LARGE, THINLY SLICED CLOVE OF GARLIC OVER

THE TOMATOES FOR A ZESTY FLAVOR.

3 thick slices of tomatoes
½ tsp sugar
juice of ½ lemon
1–2 tsp olive oil
2 thick slices of wholegrain bread, lightly toasted
½ small red onion, sliced into thin rings
*handful of fresh flat-leaf parsley or basil,
stems included*
freshly ground black pepper, to taste

1 Preheat the broiler, and line the pan with foil. Sprinkle the tomato with the sugar, and broil them on one side for 4–5 minutes, until softened and starting to brown.

2 Mix together the lemon juice and oil, then spoon this over a slice of the toasted bread. Arrange the tomatoes on the bread, and top with the onion and parsley. Season, cover with the other slice of toasted bread, and press down well before serving.

VARIATION

Eggplant Sandwich Brush a few slices of eggplant with 1 tsp olive oil, then place them under a hot broiler for 4–5 minutes, until softened and starting to brown. Combine ½ clove of crushed garlic with the lemon juice, and pour this over a slice of the toasted bread. Lay the eggplant slices on top of the bread. Finish as specified in step 2, above.

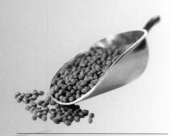

STEAMED DAHL DUMPLINGS WITH YOGURT SAUCE

THESE FLUFFY DUMPLINGS ARE SURPRISINGLY LOW IN FAT, AND MAKE A NUTRITIOUS LIGHT MEAL OR APPETIZER. SERVE THEM WITH A MIXED GREEN SALAD AND CHAPATTI OR OTHER, SIMILAR FLAT BREAD.

½ cup (75g) dried mung beans, soaked overnight, rinsed, and drained
⅓ cup (50g) dried chick-peas, soaked overnight, rinsed, and drained
2 egg whites
1 red chili, deseeded and finely chopped
3–4 tbsp chopped fresh cilantro
½ tsp cumin seeds, roasted in a dry frying pan
1 tsp baking powder
freshly ground black pepper, to taste

FOR THE SAUCE
1 cup (250ml) fat-free plain yogurt
juice of 1 lemon and ½ tsp finely grated peel
2 tbsp chopped fresh cilantro or mint, plus extra, to garnish

1 Place the mung beans, chick-peas, and egg whites in a food processor, and mix until smooth. Add the chili, cilantro, cumin, baking powder, and seasoning, then process until the mixture forms a batter-like consistency. (If the mixture is too soft, add a little flour.)

2 Line the bottom of a steamer with muslin or baking parchment. If using the latter, pierce a few holes with a thin skewer to allow the steam to penetrate. Form dumplings from tablespoonfuls of the batter mixture and place them in the steamer. Cover, and cook them for about 10 minutes, or until just firm.

3 To make the sauce, mix together all the ingredients, then pour it over the hot dumplings. Leave the sauce to soak into the dumplings for about 15 minutes. Serve either chilled or at room temperature, sprinkled with the remaining cilantro.

✳ STAR INGREDIENT
Beans are low in fat and provide valuable amounts of soluble fiber. This has been shown to help reduce cholesterol levels in the blood.

EACH SERVING PROVIDES:

○ Calories 130

○ Total Fat 1g
   Saturated Fat <1g
   Polyunsaturated Fat <1g
   Monounsaturated Fat 0g

○ Cholesterol 2mg

○ Sodium 205mg

○ Carbohydrate 20g
   Fiber 1g

○ Protein 12g

PREPARATION TIP
These dumplings do not keep well and are best eaten soon after cooking.

Preparation Time: 20 minutes, plus 15 minutes resting
Serves: 4

FRESH VEGETABLE PATTIES

1¼ cups (100g) broccoli florets
½ cup (100g) carrots, chopped
4 scallions, chopped
2 egg whites
4–5 tbsp flour

1 tsp baking powder
3–4 tbsp chopped fresh parsley or mint
freshly ground black pepper,
to taste
1 tbsp oil, for greasing

1 Place the vegetables in a food processor, then mix until finely chopped. Add the egg whites and blend, then mix in the remaining ingredients, except the oil. Cover, and refrigerate for 20 minutes.

2 Heat non-stick pan or a lightly oiled griddle. Place tablespoonfuls of the mixture on the pan, and with a small spatula spread into round patties. Cook the them for about 3 minutes on each side, until golden.

BULGAR PILAF WITH SPINACH

BULGAR IS PROBABLY ONE OF THE MOST ANCIENT "FAST FOODS".

IT IS EASY TO PREPARE, AND AN EXCELLENT AND NUTRITIOUS

ALTERNATIVE TO RICE OR COUSCOUS.

2 tbsp olive oil
1 small onion, chopped
1⅓ cups (250g) bulgar
2½ cups (600ml) boiling water
16 cups (500g) spinach, coarsely chopped
freshly ground black pepper, to taste
juice of 1 lemon

1 Heat the oil in a frying pan, then add the onion, and sauté for 5 minutes, until softened. Add the bulgar and sauté, stirring frequently, for 5 minutes, or until the grains look toasted.

2 Add the water and bring to a boil, then reduce the heat. Cover, and simmer for 15–20 minutes, until the water has been absorbed.

3 Steam the spinach for 2 minutes, or until wilted, then add it to the bulgar mixture. Season, then add the lemon juice. Cover, and leave the mixture to stand for 5 minutes before serving.

QUICK TOMATO & FRESH HERB PILAF

THIS IS A VARIATION OF THE CLASSIC MIDDLE EASTERN DISH

TABBOULEH. BULGAR WHEAT OR COUSCOUS CAN BE USED AS

A NUTRITIOUS ALTERNATIVE TO RICE.

4 tomatoes, diced
2 small cucumbers, diced
4 scallions, finely chopped
1 clove garlic, chopped
1 chili, seeded and finely chopped
juice of 1 lemon, or to taste
2 tbsp olive oil
small bunch of fresh mint or
flat-leaf parsley leaves, chopped
freshly ground black pepper, to taste
1 cup (200g) white rice
1¾ cups (400ml) water

1 Combine the tomatoes, cucumbers, scallions, garlic, chilli, lemon juice, half the oil, herbs, and seasoning in a bowl. Cover and leave to marinate for at least 1 hour to allow the flavors to develop.

2 Heat the remaining oil in a large, heavy-based saucepan. Add the rice, and sauté over a high heat, stirring constantly, for 3–4 minutes, until the rice starts to change color.

3 Add the water and bring to a rapid boil. Reduce the heat to minimum, cover, and simmer for 15 minutes, or until the rice is tender and the water has been absorbed. Leave the rice to stand for 5 minutes.

4 To serve, arrange the marinated tomato and cucumber salad on top of the cooked rice. Alternatively, mix the salad into the rice, and gently heat through before serving.

EACH SERVING PROVIDES:

- ○ Calories 270
- ○ Total Fat 8g
  Saturated Fat 1g
  Polyunsaturated Fat 1g
  Monounsaturated Fat 6g
- ○ Cholesterol 0mg
- ○ Sodium 9mg
- ○ Carbohydrate 44g
  Fiber 1g
- ○ Protein 5g

PREPARATION TIPS
Brown rice can be used instead of white. Add a little extra water and cook for 30–40 minutes, until tender. To reduce the fat content of the dish, steam or boil the rice rather than frying it.

Preparation Time: 25 minutes, plus 1 hour marinating and 5 minutes standing
Serves: 4

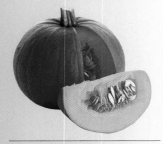

PUMPKIN RISOTTO

FOR A DECORATIVE DINNER PARTY DISH, SERVE THIS LIGHT AND FRAGRANT RISOTTO IN A SCOOPED-OUT PUMPKIN SHELL. YOU COULD USE BUTTERNUT SQUASH INSTEAD OF PUMPTKIN, WITH A TEASPOON OF CINNAMON OR NUTMEG ADDED.

✳ STAR INGREDIENT

Pumpkin is rich in vitamin C, beta-carotene, and fiber.

EACH SERVING PROVIDES:

- Calories 360
- Total Fat 9g
  Saturated Fat 1g
  Polyunsaturated Fat 1g
  Monounsaturated Fat 6g
- Cholesterol 0mg
- Sodium 230mg
- Carbohydrate 61g
  Fiber 2g
- Protein 7g

SERVING TIP

If you wish to serve the risotto in a pumpkin shell, scoop out the seeds and most of the flesh from 4 small pumpkins before filling them with the risotto.

Preparation Time: 35 minutes
Serves: 4

1lb (500g) canned, unsweetened pumpkin
2 tbsp olive oil
1 onion, finely chopped
1¼ cups (250g) arborio rice
⅓ cup (50g) golden raisins, soaked in hot water
for 20 minutes
4½ cups (1 liter) hot chicken or vegetable stock
(see pages 118–19)
juice and grated zest of 1 lemon
freshly ground black pepper, to taste
3 tbsp chopped fresh mint or flat-leaf parsley
2 tbsp pumpkin seeds, lightly roasted
in a dry skillet (optional)

1 Heat the oil in a large saucepan. Add the onion and fry for 4–5 minutes, until softened. Stir in the rice and cook for 2 minutes, until the rice is coated in the oil. Mix in the golden raisins.

2 Add about a third of the stock, reduce the heat, and simmer for 4–5 minutes, stirring frequently, until the liquid has been absorbed. Add half of the remaining stock, and simmer for 4–5 minutes, stirring frequently, until the liquid has been absorbed.

3 Add the remaining stock and the pumpkin, then simmer for a further 5–10 minutes, until the rice is creamy and tender but still retains a slight bite. Stir in the lemon juice and half of the zest, and seasoning.

4 Sprinkle the mint, pumpkin seeds, if using, and remaining lemon zest over the top of the risotto before serving.

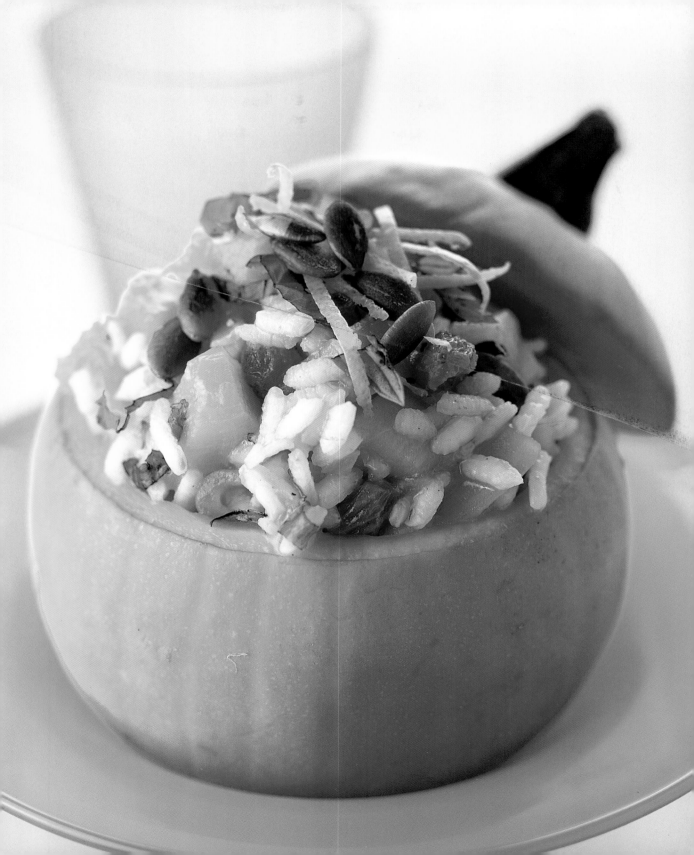

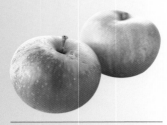

✶ STAR INGREDIENT
Apples are rich in soluble fiber and pectin, both of which may help to lower blood cholesterol levels.

EACH SERVING PROVIDES:

○ Calories 370

○ Total Fat 10g
  Saturated Fat 2g
  Polyunsaturated Fat 2g
  Monounsaturated Fat 6g

○ Cholesterol 0mg

○ Sodium 132mg

○ Carbohydrate 66g
  Fiber 4g

○ Protein 8g

PREPARATION TIP
To bake: preheat the oven to 400°F (200°C). Follow step 1, then add the apple and peas and increase the stock or water to 2½ cups (600ml). Place the pilaf in an ovenproof dish and bake, covered, for 15 minutes. Remove the lid and bake for a further 20 minutes, until the liquid has been absorbed and the rice is tender.

Preparation Time: 50 minutes, plus 5 minutes standing
Serves: 4

VEGETABLE RISOTTO

THIS SIMPLIFIED VERSION OF RISOTTO IS DELICIOUS TOPPED WITH A SPOONFUL OF PLAIN YOGURT. FOR A MORE SUBSTANTIAL MAIN COURSE, ADD SLICES OF SKINNED, ROASTED, OR BROILED CHICKEN BREAST OR FISH.

2 tbsp olive oil
1 onion, finely chopped
2 cloves garlic, finely chopped
2 carrots, grated
1¼ cups (250g) long-grain rice
1 small dessert apple, unpeeled, cored,
and finely chopped
1 cup (125g) shelled garden or frozen peas
2¼ cups (500ml) vegetable stock (see page 118) or water
a few sprigs of fresh thyme (optional)
1 tsp finely grated lemon peel (optional)
freshly ground black pepper, to taste

❶ Heat the oil in a heavy-based saucepan with a lid. Add the onion, garlic, and carrots, then sauté for 8–10 minutes, until browned. Add the rice and fry, stirring, for 1 minute, until it is coated in the oil mixture.

❷ Add the apple, peas, and stock. Bring to a boil, then reduce the heat to minimum and cover the pan with a tight-fitting lid. Simmer gently for about 20–25 minutes, or until the rice is tender and the water has been absorbed.

❸ Add the thyme and lemon peel, if using, and season. Fluff up the rice with a fork, and leave to stand, covered, for 5 minutes before serving.

VARIATION
Pineapple Vegetable Risotto Replace the apples with 5oz (150g) pineapple, cored and chopped, and 2½ teaspoons (30g) golden raisins, soaked in hot water for 20 minutes.

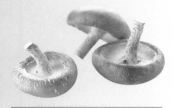

ORIENTAL MUSHROOM RISOTTO

INCORPORATING CREAMY, ITALIAN ARBORIO RICE AND ORIENTAL

SHIITAKE MUSHROOMS, THIS RECIPE COMBINES THE DELICIOUS

FLAVORS OF EAST AND WEST. SERVE THIS DISH WITH

A MIXED GREEN SALAD.

2 tbsp sunflower oil
1 small onion, finely chopped
2 cloves garlic, chopped
¾in (1.5cm) piece fresh ginger, finely shredded
1½ cups (125g) shiitake mushrooms, stems discarded,
and caps thickly sliced
1½ cups (125g) cremini mushrooms, sliced
1 cup (250ml) dry white wine
1¼ cups (250g) arborio rice
3 cups (750ml) hot chicken or vegetable stock
(see pages 118–19)
freshly ground black pepper, to taste
1 tbsp chopped fresh thyme or
2 tbsp chopped fresh flat-leaf parsley
shavings of Parmesan, to garnish (optional)

1 Heat the oil in a large, heavy-based saucepan, then add the onion, garlic, and ginger. Sauté for 4–5 minutes, until the onion starts to brown.

2 Add all the mushrooms and sauté for 4–5 minutes, until the mushrooms soften and start to exude liquid. Add the white wine and bring to a boil. Reduce the heat and simmer, uncovered, for 10 minutes, or until most of the liquid has evaporated.

3 Add the rice, and stir for about 1 minute, or until the rice is coated in the mushroom mixture. Add about a third of the stock and simmer for 5–6 minutes, stirring occasionally, until the liquid has been absorbed. Add half of the remaining stock and cook, stirring frequently, until the liquid has been absorbed.

4 Add the remaining stock and cook for a further 5–6 minutes, until the rice is creamy and tender but still firm to the bite. Season, then sprinkle with the thyme and Parmesan, if using, before serving.

✴ STAR INGREDIENT
Shiitake and other oriental mushrooms have been found to lower levels of harmful cholesterol in the body.

EACH SERVING PROVIDES:

○ Calories 430

○ Total Fat 9g
  Saturated Fat 1g
  Polyunsaturated Fat 5g
  Monounsaturated Fat 2g

○ Cholesterol 0mg

○ Sodium 180mg

○ Carbohydrate 77g
  Fiber 1g

○ Protein 15g

PREPARATION TIP
If you cannot find fresh shiitake mushrooms, use dried instead. Rehydrate ½ cup (30g) dried mushrooms in hot water for 30 minutes. Remove and discard the stems and use the mushrooms as specified.

Preparation Time: 40 minutes
Serves: 4

EGGPLANT & TOMATO WITH PASTA

PASTA IS A CONVENIENT AND VERSATILE LOW FAT FOOD. CHOOSE FROM THE WIDE RANGE OF PASTA SHAPES NOW AVAILABLE TO ACCOMPANY THE RICH, AROMATIC TOMATO SAUCE. SERVE THIS DISH WITH A SALAD.

2 tbsp olive oil
1 large onion, chopped
4 cloves garlic, chopped
1 small (250g) eggplant, cut into ½in (1cm) cubes
1 tbsp reduced-salt soy sauce
13oz (400g) canned, crushed, unsalted tomatoes
*3–4 (250g) plum tomatoes, skinned, seeded,
and chopped*
2 tbsp chopped fresh thyme or oregano
*2½ cups (300g) pasta shapes, such as riccioli,
fusilli, or conchiglie*
freshly ground black pepper, to taste
*handful of chopped fresh flat-leaf parsley,
to garnish*

1 Heat the oil in a large, heavy-based saucepan, then add the onion and garlic. Sauté for 5–8 minutes, until the onion has softened. Add the eggplant and cook for another 5 minutes, or until it has softened slightly. If the mixture becomes too dry, add 1–2 tablespoons of water.

2 Add the soy sauce and cook for 1–2 minutes, stirring. Add the canned tomatoes, breaking down any large lumps with the back of a spoon. Cover, and cook for about 20 minutes, or until the eggplant is soft and tender. Add the fresh tomatoes and thyme, and simmer for a further 2 minutes to heat through.

3 While the sauce is cooking, prepare the pasta following the manufacturer's instructions. Season the sauce, and serve with the pasta. Sprinkle with the parsley before serving.

✶ STAR INGREDIENT
Tomatoes are a central part of Mediterranean cooking, which is widely recognized as being beneficial for the heart.

EACH SERVING PROVIDES:

○ Calories 380

○ Total Fat 10g
Saturated Fat 1g
Polyunsaturated Fat 2g
Monounsaturated Fat 6g

○ Cholesterol 0mg

○ Sodium 287mg

○ Carbohydrate 67g
Fiber 2g

○ Protein 12g

PREPARATION TIP
Avoid peeling the eggplant, since the skin helps to retain the shape of the cubes and enhances the appearance of the dish.

Preparation Time: 45 minutes
Serves: 4

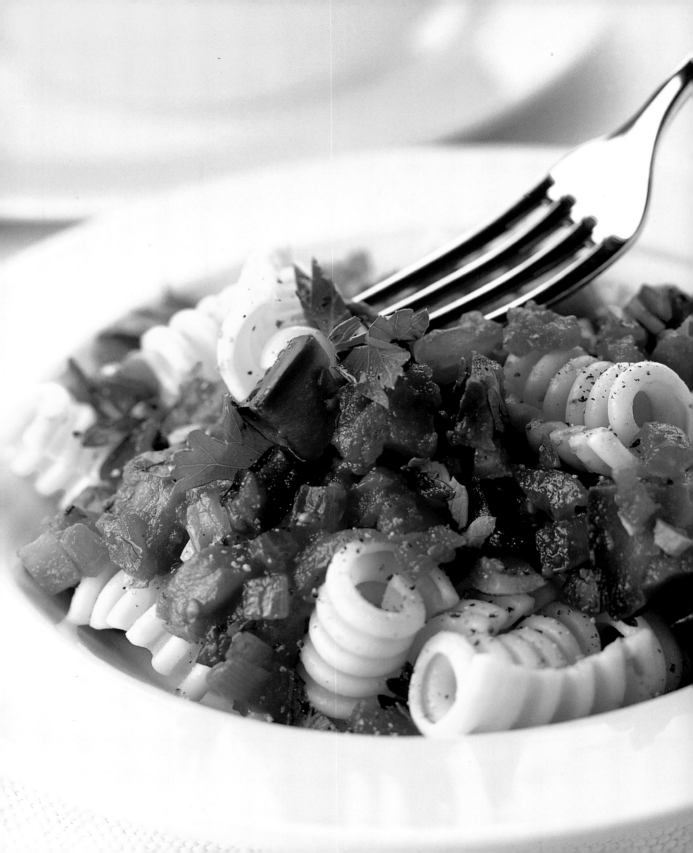

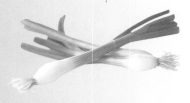

COTTAGE CHEESE & FRESH HERBS WITH PASTA

VIRTUALLY FAT-FREE, COTTAGE CHEESE CAN BE A STAPLE IN THE HEART
HEALTHY KITCHEN. TANGY, CREAMY, AND VERSATILE, IT ALSO ADDS
TEXTURE AND MOISTURE TO SAUCES, SALADS, AND SANDWICHES.

10oz (300g) fusilli
1 tbsp olive oil
1 cup (250g) 1 percent low fat or fat-free cottage cheese
4 scallions, finely chopped
small bunch of fresh flat-leaf parsley,
coarsely chopped
freshly ground black pepper, to taste

1 Cook the pasta following the manufacturer's instructions, then drain.

2 Heat the oil in a saucepan, then add the pasta, tossing until it is coated in the oil. Add the remaining ingredients, reserving a little of the parsley to garnish, and mix well. Heat through, and serve sprinkled with the reserved parsley.

VARIATION

Garlic and Fresh Herbs with Pasta Replace the cottage cheese with 1 tablespoon of olive oil and 1 crushed clove of garlic.

✴ STAR INGREDIENT
The onion family has been found to have both cleansing and healing properties, including the reduction of cholesterol levels in the blood.

EACH SERVING PROVIDES:

○ Calories 340

○ Total Fat 6g
  Saturated Fat 1g
  Polyunsaturated Fat 1g
  Monounsaturated Fat 3g

○ Cholesterol 3mg

○ Sodium 243mg

○ Carbohydrate 58g
  Fiber g

○ Protein 18g

PREPARATION TIP
This dish is equally delicious served cold. Stir the cheese and the rest of the ingredients into the warm pasta. Leave to cool, then chill before serving.

Preparation Time: 20 minutes
Serves: 4

TAGLIATELLE WITH TUNA SAUCE

VERSATILE AS WELL AS CONVENIENT, CANNED TUNA IS A USEFUL

STANDBY, BUT BE SURE TO BUY TUNA IN SPRING WATER RATHER

THAN IN OIL, AND RINSE WITH WATER. SERVE THIS DISH

WITH A GREEN SALAD.

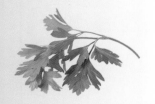

★ STAR INGREDIENT
Parsley contains rich amounts of the antioxidants vitamin C and beta-carotene, as well as iron and calcium.

EACH SERVING PROVIDES:

○ Calories 420

○ Total Fat 10g
  Saturated Fat 1g
  Polyunsaturated Fat 1g
  Monounsaturated Fat 6g

○ Cholesterol 26mg

○ Sodium 200mg

○ Carbohydrate 65g
  Fiber 5g

○ Protein 23g

PREPARATION TIP
To reduce the salt content of capers, soak them in warm water for 20 minutes, then drain and rinse well.

Preparation Time: 50 minutes
Serves: 4

---

2 tbsp olive oil
1 tsp fennel seeds (optional)
1 large onion, chopped
3 cloves garlic, chopped
4 medium (500g) tomatoes, skinned, deseeded, and chopped
2 tbsp tomato purée, diluted in ½ cup (100ml)
red or white wine, stock
(see pages 118–19), or water
bouquet garni, made up of a few sprigs
of fresh thyme, fennel leaves, sprig of parsley,
and 2 strips of grated lemon peel
10oz (300g) tagliatelle
7oz (200g) canned tuna in spring water,
drained, rinsed, and flaked
2 tsp capers, rinsed and coarsely chopped
(left whole, if small)
3 tbsp chopped fresh parsley or
2 tbsp fresh lemon thyme or tarragon
freshly ground black pepper, to taste

1 Heat the oil in a large skillet. Add the fennel seeds, if using, and cook for 2–3 minutes, or until they release a spicy aroma. Add the onion and garlic, then cook for 5 minutes, or until the onion has softened. If the mixture becomes too dry, add 1–2 tablespoons of water.

2 Add the tomatoes, the tomato purée mixture, and the bouquet garni. Bring to a boil, reduce the heat, and simmer for about 30 minutes, or until most of the liquid has evaporated.

3 Cook the pasta following the manufacturer's instructions, then drain.

4 Add the tuna, capers, and parsley to the tomato sauce. Season, and continue to cook for 2–3 minutes to allow the flavors to develop. Mix the sauce into the cooked tagliatelle before serving.

BAKED COD WITH TOMATO & PEPPER SALSA

TOMATOES, PEPPERS, AND PARSLEY ADD TO THE APPEARANCE AND NUTRITIONAL VALUE OF THIS EASY DISH. SERVE IT WITH A VEGETABLE SUCH AS GREEN BEANS AND MEDITERRANEAN BEAN SOUP (*SEE PAGE 42*).

juice of 2 lemons, and grated peel of 1, plus extra, to garnish
4 cod or haddock steaks, each about 6oz (175g)
2 tbsp olive oil
freshly ground black pepper, to taste

FOR THE SALSA
4 plum tomatoes, peeled, seeded, and finely chopped
1 yellow or green pepper, cored, seeded, and finely chopped
1 celery stick, finely chopped
1 onion, finely chopped
1–2 green chilies, seeded and finely chopped
1 clove garlic, minced
small bunch of fresh flat-leaf parsley, finely chopped

1 Place the lemon juice and grated peel in a shallow dish, then add the fish, turning once to coat both sides. Cover, and refrigerate for 30 minutes.

2 Mix together the salsa ingredients in a bowl, reserving some parsley.

3 Preheat the oven to 425°F (220°C). Brush a baking dish with a little of the oil, then arrange the fish on it. Spoon the salsa over the steaks and season. Sprinkle with the marinade and the remaining oil. Bake for 20 minutes, until tender. Garnish with grated lemon peel and parsley.

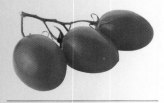

✳ STAR INGREDIENT
Tomatoes are a good source of vitamins E and C, and also contain the antioxidant lycopene, which protects against heart disease.

EACH SERVING PROVIDES:

- ○ Calories 230
- ○ Total Fat 9g
  Saturated Fat 1g
  Polyunsaturated Fat 1g
  Monounsaturated Fat 6g
- ○ Cholesterol 68mg
- ○ Sodium 159mg
- ○ Carbohydrate 6g
  Fiber 2g
- ○ Protein 31g

PREPARATION TIP
Other fish, such as haddock, halibut, or trout, can be used instead of cod.

Preparation Time: 40 minutes, plus 30 minutes marinating
Serves: 4

MAIN MEALS

These innovative and inspiring recipes incorporate all the nutritional prerequisites necessary for a healthy heart and body. Serve them with fresh salads, steamed vegetables, or simple grain dishes for a well-balanced meal.

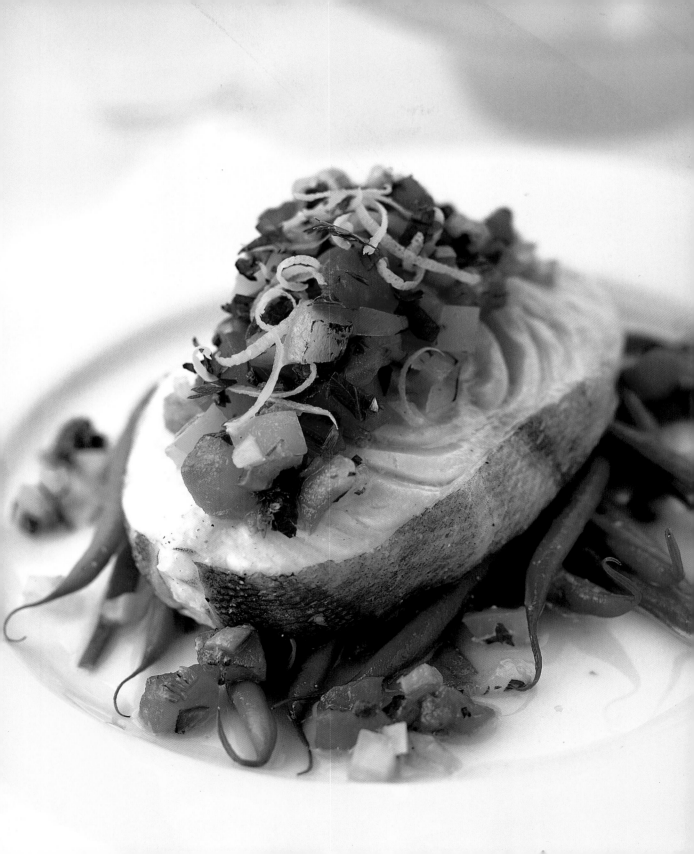

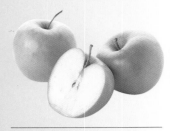

★ STAR INGREDIENT
Apple skin contains quercetin, which may protect against heart disease, as well as pectin, which is believed to help lower blood-cholesterol levels.

EACH SERVING PROVIDES:

○ Calories 295

○ Total Fat 9g
 Saturated Fat 1g
 Polyunsaturated Fat 2g
 Monounsaturated Fat 5g

○ Cholesterol 61mg

○ Sodium 113mg

○ Carbohydrate 12g
 Fiber 3g

○ Protein 39g

PREPARATION TIP
If halibut is unavailable, other firm fish, such as monkfish, shark, or cod, can be used.

Preparation Time: 40 minutes, plus 30 minutes marinating
Serves: 4

BAKED HALIBUT WITH APPLES

HALIBUT IS A LEAN, FIRM FISH, WHICH WHEN BAKED WITH APPLES AND WHITE WINE, RETAINS ITS MOIST TEXTURE AND VALUABLE NUTRIENTS. THIS LIGHT DISH MAY BE SERVED WITH QUICK TOMATO & FRESH HERB PILAF (*SEE PAGE 51*) AND STEAMED BROCCOLI OR GREEN BEANS.

*juice and grated peel of 1 lemon, or juice of 2 limes
and grated peel of 1 lime
4 halibut steaks, each about 6oz (175g)
1½ tbsp olive oil
2 tart apples, such as Granny Smiths, cored
and sliced into ¼in (5mm) rings
2 onions, thinly sliced
1 large red pepper, cored, seeded, and sliced into thin rings
1–2 red or green chilies, seeded and thinly sliced (optional)
4 tbsp chopped fresh flat-leaf parsley or dill
freshly ground black pepper, to taste
4 tbsp dry white wine*

1 Place the lemon juice and grated peel in a shallow dish, then add the fish, turning it in the juice to coat both sides. Cover, and refrigerate for 30 minutes.

2 Preheat the oven to 425° F (220°C). Brush a baking dish with a little of the oil. Arrange half the apples in the bottom of the dish, then top with half the onions and pepper.

3 Place the fish on top, reserving the marinade, and sprinkle with the chilies, if using, and half the parsley. Repeat with another layer of the onions and pepper slices, and finally the apples, then season.

4 Pour the reserved marinade, wine, and remaining oil over the apples. Bake for 15–20 minutes, basting the fish occasionally with some of the juices. Remove from the oven and cool briefly. Scatter the rest of the parsley on top before serving.

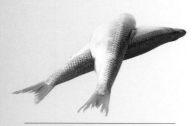

STUFFED HERRINGS

LIKE OTHER OILY FISH, HERRINGS ARE RICH IN OMEGA-3 FATTY ACIDS, WHICH LOWER THE RISK OF HEART DISEASE. THIS DISH IS BASED ON A CLASSIC BRITISH RECIPE AND IS BEST SERVED WITH A SALAD AND NEW POTATOES.

1 onion, thinly sliced
4 herrings, each about 7½oz (225g),
heads removed, gutted, and boned
4 tsp mustard
4 tsp brown sugar
4 tbsp chopped fresh parsley
1 bay leaf
10 black peppercorns
4 cloves
1–2 small dried chilies (optional)
½ cup (100ml) dry white wine
3 tbsp white wine vinegar

1 Preheat the oven to 400°F (200°C). Place the onion in a small bowl, and cover with boiling water. Soak for 1 minute, then drain. Refresh the onion in cold water, then drain well and set aside.

2 Dry the herrings with paper towels, and open them out on a board, skin-side down. Spread the mustard over the flesh, and sprinkle with the sugar. Divide the prepared onion between the herrings, and sprinkle with the parsley. Roll up the herrings, head-end first, to form thick rolls, and secure each one with a wooden skewer.

3 Arrange the fish rolls in a baking dish, then scatter over the bay leaf and spices. Pour the wine and vinegar over the fish, then season. Cover with foil, and bake for 25 minutes.

4 Increase the heat to 450°F (230°C). Remove the foil and bake, basting the fish frequently with the juices, for a further 10–15 minutes, until the herrings are tender and the juices have reduced. Allow to stand for about 10 minutes before serving.

✳ STAR INGREDIENT

Herrings contain omega-3 fatty acids, which may help to lower cholesterol levels in the body. Along with reducing the risk of heart attacks, these beneficial oils may lower blood pressure.

EACH SERVING PROVIDES:

○ Calories 270

○ Total Fat 15g
  Saturated Fat 4g
  Polyunsaturated Fat 3g
  Monounsaturated Fat 7g

○ Cholesterol 55mg

○ Sodium 139mg

○ Carbohydrate 8g
  Fiber 1g

○ Protein 21g

SERVING TIP

This dish is delicious cold and can be made the day before it is served. Store, covered, in the refrigerator and remove an hour before serving. Catfish or shrimp can be substituted for the herring.

Preparation Time: 60 minutes, plus 10 minutes standing
Serves: 4

BROILED MACKEREL WITH CITRUS SALSA

MACKEREL PLAYS AN IMPORTANT PART IN THE HEALTHY HEART
DIET AS IT CONTAINS VALUABLE OMEGA-3 FATTY ACIDS, WHICH HELP
TO LOWER CHOLESTEROL LEVELS. SERVE THIS DISH WITH
A COMBINATION OF WILD AND WHITE RICE.

4 mackerel fillets, each about 3½oz (100g)
juice of 1 lemon and 1 tsp grated peel
2 tsp paprika (optional)
fresh mint leaves, to garnish

FOR THE SALSA
2 oranges, segmented and cut into ½in (1cm) pieces
2 large lemons, segmented and cut into ½in (1cm) pieces
½–1 tsp dried chili flakes
1 tbsp chopped fresh mint or parsley
freshly ground black pepper, to taste

1 Mix together the salsa ingredients in a bowl. Cover, and refrigerate for at least an hour to allow the flavors to develop.

2 Place the fish in a shallow dish and spoon over the lemon juice and grated peel, rubbing them into the flesh. Cover, and refrigerate for 30 minutes.

3 Heat the broiler to high. Sprinkle the paprika, if using, over each fillet and broil the fish for 3–4 minutes on each side, until tender. Serve with the citrus salsa and garnish with the mint leaves.

VARIATION
Baked Mackerel Preheat the oven to 425°F (220°C). Follow steps 1 and 2, above, then place the fish in a lightly oiled baking dish and sprinkle the paprika over each fillet. Spoon the citrus salsa over the fillets. Bake for 10–15 minutes, until the fish is tender. Serve, garnished with the mint leaves. Pompano, bluefish, or Chilean sea bass can be used instead of mackerel.

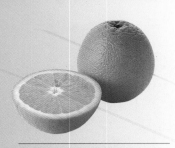

★ STAR INGREDIENT
Oranges are one of the best-known sources of vitamin C, which may help to prevent cell damage.

EACH SERVING PROVIDES:

○ Calories 270

○ Total Fat 17g
  Saturated Fat 4g
  Polyunsaturated Fat 4g
  Monounsaturated Fat 8g

○ Cholesterol 54mg

○ Sodium 86mg

○ Carbohydrate 10g
  Fiber 1g

○ Protein 21g

PREPARATION TIP
The paprika adds a spicy flavor to the mackerel fillets but can be omitted if preferred.

Preparation Time: 30 minutes, plus 1 hour marinating
Serves: 4

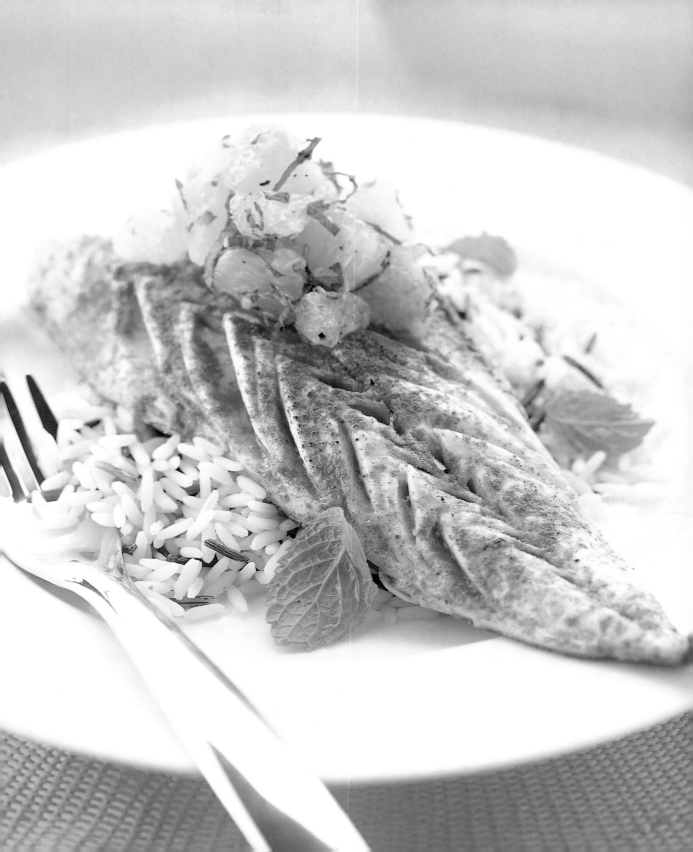

BROILED SARDINES WITH CHILI TOMATO SALSA

FRESH SARDINES ARE PACKED WITH FLAVOR AND FULL OF HEALTHY OMEGA-3 FATTY ACIDS, WHICH HELP LOWER BLOOD-CHOLESTEROL LEVELS, REDUCING THE RISK OF HEART DISEASE. THE PIQUANT CHILI TOMATO SALSA ADDS A REFRESHING TANG.

4 sardines, each about 6oz (175g), gutted and boned
juice and grated peel of 1 lemon

FOR THE SALSA
4 plum tomatoes, peeled, seeded, and finely chopped
1 small red or white onion, finely chopped
1–2 cloves garlic, crushed
1–2 green chilies, seeded and finely chopped
small bunch of fresh flat-leaf parsley, dill, or mint, chopped
juice of 1 lemon and ½ tsp grated peel
freshly ground black pepper, to taste

1 Cut three deep slashes down the sides of each sardine. Place the fish in a shallow dish, and sprinkle with the lemon juice and grated peel, rubbing them into the skin and flesh. Cover, and refrigerate for 30 minutes.

2 Mix together the salsa ingredients in a bowl. Cover, and refrigerate for 30 minutes to allow the flavors to develop.

3 Preheat the broiler. Broil the sardines for 3–4 minutes on each side, until tender and browned. Serve with the salsa.

VARIATION
Marinated Sardines Mix together 1 tablespoon reduced-salt soy sauce, juice of 1 lime or lemon, plus 1 teaspoon grated peel, 1 stick of lemongrass, peeled and finely chopped, 3 scallions, finely shredded, and 5 tablespoons rice wine or dry sherry. Follow step 3, above, then pour the marinade over the hot, broiled sardines. Allow to cool and serve with the Chili Tomato Salsa.

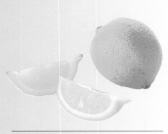

✳ STAR INGREDIENT
Like other citrus fruit, lemons are rich in vitamin C and potassium, which regulates blood pressure. The pectin in lemons, found mainly in the skin around each segment, is reputed to help reduce blood-cholesterol levels.

EACH SERVING PROVIDES:

○ Calories 225

○ Total Fat 11g
Saturated Fat 3g
Polyunsaturated Fat 4g
Monounsaturated Fat 3g

○ Cholesterol 105mg

○ Sodium 156mg

○ Carbohydrate 3g
Fiber 1g

○ Protein 28g

SERVING TIP
This dish is best served simply with slices of wholewheat or seeded bread.

Preparation Time: 20 minutes, plus 30 minutes marinating
Serves: 4

EACH SERVING PROVIDES:

○ Calories 250

○ Total Fat 1g
   Saturated Fat 2g
   Polyunsaturated Fat 3g
   Monounsaturated Fat 6g

○ Cholesterol 32mg

○ Sodium 96mg

○ Carbohydrate 19g
   Fiber 1g

○ Protein 20g

PREPARATION TIPS

Other types of fish can be used but it is important to select two varieties: an oily fish, such as tuna or salmon; and a lean white fish, such as bream, halibut or cod. If you have a mincer, use this instead of a food processor.

Preparation Time: 25 minutes, plus 30 minutes chilling
Serves: 4

BROILED FISH CAKES WITH CUCUMBER SALSA

THESE DELICIOUS, LIGHTLY SPICED FISH CAKES ARE A NUTRITIOUS COMBINATION OF WHITE AND OILY FISH. SERVE THEM WITH NEW POTATOES, RICE, OR PASTA FOR A SATISFYING MAIN COURSE.

5oz (150g) mackerel fillets, skinned and cut into pieces
7oz (200g) hake fillets, skinned and cut into pieces
4 scallions, finely chopped
1 red chili, seeded and finely chopped
1 clove garlic, crushed
100g (3½oz) cooked rice or barley
4 tbsp matzo meal or breadcrumbs
1 egg white
1 tsp finely grated lemon peel
freshly ground black pepper, to taste
1 tbsp olive oil

FOR THE SALSA
1 cucumber, seeded and finely chopped
1 clove garlic, crushed
1–2 chilies, seeded and finely chopped
1 stick of lemongrass, peeled and finely chopped
juice of 2 lemons, plus ½ tsp grated peel
2 tbsp chopped fresh cilantro

1 Mix together the ingredients for the salsa in a bowl. Cover, and refrigerate for 30 minutes to allow the flavors to develop.

2 Place the fish in a food processor, and process until finely chopped but not puréed. Mix with the remaining ingredients, except the oil, in a bowl. Cover, and refrigerate for 30 minutes. Divide the mixture into 8 portions and, using your hands, shape each portion into a flat cake.

3 Preheat the broiler. Brush the cakes with the oil and broil for about 5 minutes on each side, until golden. (Alternatively, pan broil the cakes in a non-stick frying pan for the same length of time.) Serve with the salsa.

CHINESE STEAMED SEA BASS

THIS IS A CLASSIC, CHINESE-INSPIRED DISH THAT MAKES A SIMPLE, YET ATTRACTIVE MAIN COURSE FOR A DINNER PARTY. FLAVORED WITH GINGER, GARLIC, AND SCALLIONS, THE DISH IS EXCELLENT SERVED WITH NOODLES OR RICE.

4 sea bass fillets, each about 6oz (175g)
4 scallions, sliced into fine strips
1 carrot, sliced into fine strips
1in (2.5cm) piece of fresh ginger, sliced into fine strips
1 mild red chili, seeded and sliced into fine strips
2 tsp reduced-salt soy sauce
1 tbsp mirin
2 tsp sake or dry sherry
2 tbsp sesame seeds, toasted in a dry frying pan

1 Place the fish on a plate, in a steamer or toaster oven. Arrange the vegetables, ginger, and chili on top of each fillet, then spoon over the soy sauce, mirin, and sake. Cover, and steam for 10 minutes, or until the fish is opaque, flaky, and tender.

2 Place the fish and vegetables, with their cooking juices, on a warmed plate. Scatter the sesame seeds over the fish before serving. (The seeds can also be scattered over the accompanying noodles or rice).

VARIATION

Chinese Steamed Chicken Replace the sea bass with 4 skinless, boneless chicken breasts, each about 4oz (125g), sliced into strips, and the carrot with 1 red pepper, deseeded and sliced into strips. Place the chicken on a plate, in a steamer. Cover and steam for 10 minutes. Remove from the heat and arrange the vegetables on top of the chicken, then spoon over the soy sauce, mirin, and sake. Cover, and steam for 5–10 minutes, until the chicken and vegetables are tender. To serve the chicken, follow step 2, above.

★ STAR INGREDIENT
Sea bass is naturally low in fat and high in iodine, protein, and selenium. It also contains useful amounts of vitamin E.

EACH SERVING PROVIDES:

○ Calories 235

○ Total Fat 9g
Saturated Fat 1g
Polyunsaturated Fat 4g
Monounsaturated Fat 3g

○ Cholesterol 140mg

○ Sodium 236mg

○ Carbohydrate 3g
Fiber 2g

○ Protein 36g

PREPARATION TIP
To make the fish even more fragrant, add a small cinnamon stick, 2 star anise, and a finely chopped stick of lemongrass to the cooking water.

Preparation Time: 20 minutes
Serves: 4

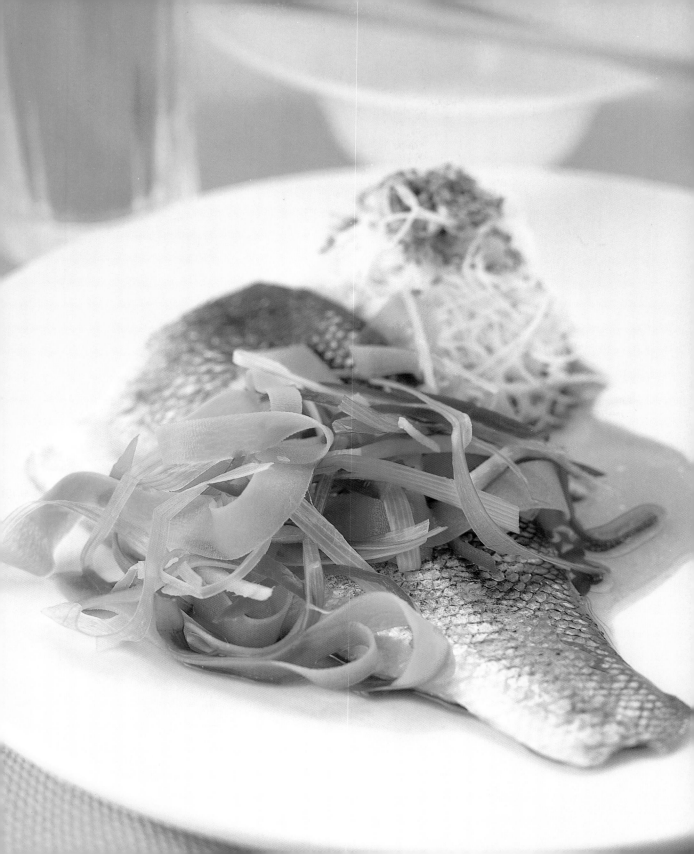

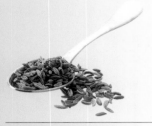

EACH SERVING PROVIDES:

○ Calories 150

○ Total Fat 5g
  Saturated Fat 1g
  Polyunsaturated Fat 3g
  Monounsaturated Fat 1g

○ Cholesterol 18mg

○ Sodium 77mg

○ Carbohydrate 4g
  Fiber 1g

○ Protein 25g

PREPARATION TIPS
Try experimenting with different
types of fish: white fish, including
cod or halibut, or fatty fish, such
as Chilean sea bass, mackerel, or
salmon, are delicious alternatives
to the monkfish. Remember to
remove the cinnamon stick and
bay leaf before serving the curry.

Preparation Time: 50 minutes
Serves: 4

MONKFISH CURRY WITH CORIANDER

MOST KINDS OF FIRM-FLESHED WHITE FISH ARE SUITABLE

FOR THIS CREAMY, KORMA-STYLE CURRY. SERVE IT WITH PLAIN RICE

AND FENNEL & RUBY GRAPEFRUIT SALAD (*SEE PAGE 92*).

1 tsp ground fennel seeds
1 tsp ground coriander
juice and grated peel of 1 lime
1lb (500g) monkfish, cut into bite-sized cubes
1 large onion, coarsely chopped
4 cloves garlic, chopped
1in (2.5cm) piece of fresh ginger, peeled and chopped
1–2 green chilies, seeded and coarsely chopped
1 tbsp sunflower oil
½ tsp fennel seeds
1in (2.5cm) piece of cinnamon stick
1 bay leaf
1¼ cups (300ml) fish or chicken stock (see pages 118–19),
or white wine
½ cup (100ml) fat-free yogurt
freshly ground black pepper, to taste
fresh cilantro, to garnish

1 Mix together the spices, lime juice, and grated peel in a dish. Add the fish, turning it in the mixture. Cover, and refrigerate for 30 minutes.

2 Place the onion, garlic, ginger, and chilies in a food processor, then process into a smooth paste. Heat the oil in a saucepan. Add the fennel seeds, cinnamon stick, and bay leaf, and cook for 1 minute over a medium heat. Add the spice paste to the pan, and cook, stirring, for about 5 minutes, or until the mixture starts to color.

3 Add the stock and cook, stirring frequently, for about 20 minutes, or until the mixture has thickened.

4 Add the fish with its marinade, then reduce the heat and simmer for 10 minutes, or until the fish is tender. Stir in the yogurt and seasoning, then heat through. Garnish with the cilantro before serving.

TEA-SMOKED SALMON

HOT-SMOKING IS A SIMPLE, TOTALLY FAT-FREE METHOD OF COOKING

THAT DOES NOT REQUIRE ANY SPECIAL EQUIPMENT AND SUITS MOST

TYPES OF FISH. THIS FRAGRANT DISH CAN BE SERVED WITH NEW

POTATOES AND ROASTED GARLIC & ZUCCHINI SALAD (*SEE PAGE 90*).

4 salmon steaks, each about 4oz (125g)
juice of ½ lemon, ¼ tsp grated peel, and 2 strips
of lemon peel
freshly ground black pepper, to taste
2 tbsp black tea leaves
4–5 star anise, crushed
1–2 cinnamon sticks, crushed
a few sprigs of fresh thyme and rosemary

1 Sprinkle the fish with the lemon juice and grated peel. Cover, and refrigerate for about 1 hour.

2 Line a large, lidded wok or saucepan with a layer of heavy-duty foil, and place the pepper, tea leaves, star anise, cinnamon, thyme, and rosemary on top. Place a wire rack inside the wok or saucepan, then arrange the fish on top. Cover tightly with the lid.

3 Place the pan over a high heat until it starts smoking. Reduce the heat to low, and smoke for 10–15 minutes, until the fish is tender. Turn off the heat and allow to cool, with the lid on, for about 5 minutes.

VARIATION

Tea-smoked Chicken Marinate 4 x 4oz (125g) skinless, boneless chicken breast halves in the lemon juice as in step 1, above, then steam the chicken for 10 minutes, until tender. Prepare the saucepan or wok as in step 2, above, substituting the chicken for the fish. Cover tightly. Follow step 3, above, cooking the chicken for 20–25 minutes, until tender and smoked.

✱ STAR INGREDIENT
Salmon is an oily fish that is rich in unsaturated fats, particularly omega-3 fatty acids, which can reduce the risk of heart disease.

EACH SERVING PROVIDES:

○ Calories 230

○ Total Fat 14g
  Saturated Fat 2g
  Polyunsaturated Fat 5g
  Monounsaturated Fat 6g

○ Cholesterol 63mg

○ Sodium 56mg

○ Carbohydrate <1g
  Fiber 0g

○ Protein 25g

PREPARATION TIP
Although any type of tea can be used, Lapsang Souchong is preferable, since it has a wonderfully smoky flavor.

Preparation Time: 25 minutes
Serves: 4

CHICKEN & PINEAPPLE CURRY

ALTHOUGH THIS RECIPE IS MADE WITH PINEAPPLE, PAPAYA IS

A SUITABLE ALTERNATIVE, SINCE THESE FRUITS CONTAIN AN ENZYME

THAT TENDERIZES MEAT, MAKING IT EASIER TO DIGEST. SERVE THIS

FRAGRANT CURRY DISH WITH PLAIN, STEAMED RICE.

1 onion, chopped
3 cloves garlic
1in (2.5cm) piece of fresh ginger, chopped
1 ripe pineapple, peeled, cored, and coarsely chopped
2–3 red chilies, seeded and chopped
2 tsp coriander seeds, ground
2 cardamom pods, ground
½ tsp ground cinnamon
1 tbsp brown sugar
1 tbsp sunflower or light olive oil, plus extra for greasing
1½ cups (375ml) water
6 skinless, boneless chicken thighs, each about 3oz (75g)
6 tbsp fat-free yogurt
3–4 tbsp fresh cilantro or dill, to garnish

1 Preheat the oven to 450°F (230°C). Arrange the onion, garlic, ginger, pineapple, and chilies in a baking dish. Spoon the spices, sugar, oil, and 4 tablespoons of the water over the onion mixture. Bake for 25 minutes, turning the mixture occasionally, until it starts to caramelize.

2 Heat a lightly oiled griddle and cook the chicken for 3–4 minutes on each side, until golden, then set aside and keep hot.

3 Transfer the pineapple mixture to a food processor, and blend into a smooth purée. Mix together the remaining water and the yogurt, then put them in a saucepan with the pineapple mixture.

4 Bring the mixture to a boil, then reduce the heat. Add the chicken and simmer, uncovered, for about 45 minutes, or until the sauce has reduced and thickened and the chicken is tender. Garnish with the cilantro before serving.

✶ STAR INGREDIENT
Chicken is a good source of low fat protein as long as the skin is removed before cooking.

EACH SERVING PROVIDES:

○ Calories 245

○ Total Fat 10g
 Saturated Fat 2g
 Polyunsaturated Fat 4g
 Monounsaturated Fat 4g

○ Cholesterol 96mg

○ Sodium 119mg

○ Carbohydrate 14g
 Fiber 1g

○ Protein 28g

PREPARATION TIP
If the sauce is too watery at the end of the cooking time, increase the heat and boil rapidly, stirring frequently, until it has thickened.

Preparation Time: 1 hour, 25 minutes
Serves: 4

TANDOORI CHICKEN

TENDER PIECES OF CHICKEN ARE MARINATED IN A COMBINATION OF

YOGURT AND SPICES IN THIS TRADITIONAL INDIAN CELEBRATION

DISH. IT MAKES A WONDERFUL, LIGHT MEAL THAT MAY BE

ACCOMPANIED BY RICE AND APPLE & CABBAGE SALAD (*SEE PAGE 98*).

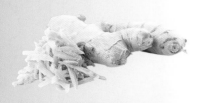

✷ STAR INGREDIENT
Ginger is a warming, aromatic spice with numerous health benefits. It can effectively relieve indigestion, stimulate circulation, and combat colds and coughs.

EACH SERVING PROVIDES:

○ Calories 245

○ Total Fat 9g
Saturated Fat 2g
Polyunsaturated Fat 2g
Monounsaturated Fat 4g

○ Cholesterol 128mg

○ Sodium 188mg

○ Carbohydrate 5g
Fiber <1g

○ Protein 41g

SERVING TIP
A good lunchtime main course, this dish may also be served cold as part of a buffet.

Preparation Time: 1 hour, 10 minutes, plus 8–12 hours marinating
Serves: 4

6 cloves garlic, chopped
2in (5cm) piece of fresh ginger, chopped
1 cup (250ml) fat-free yogurt
juice of 2 limes and grated peel of 1 lime
2 tbsp ground coriander
1 tbsp paprika
1 tbsp ground cumin
1 tbsp turmeric
1–2 tsp chili powder
1 tsp ground cardamom
8 skinless chicken thighs, each about 3oz (75g)
quartered limes, to garnish

1 Purée the garlic and ginger using a mortar or food processor, and blend into a smooth paste. Add the yogurt, lime juice and grated peel, and the rest of the spices, and blend well.

2 Prick the chicken all over with a fork. Put the chicken in a baking dish, then spoon over two-thirds of the spice paste, rubbing it well into the meat. (Reserve the rest of the spice paste.) Let it marinate, covered, for about 8–12 hours in the refrigerator.

3 Preheat the oven to 400°F (200°C). Line a baking sheet with foil. Put the marinated chicken on a rack placed over the lined baking sheet. Spread the reserved spice paste over the chicken, and bake for 45–60 minutes, until the chicken is tender. Serve with the lime quarters.

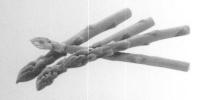

✴ STAR INGREDIENT
Asparagus is a rich source of folate, which is thought to help protect against heart disease.

EACH SERVING PROVIDES:

○ Calories 230

○ Total Fat 10g
Saturated Fat 2g
Polyunsaturated Fat 3g
Monounsaturated Fat 4g

○ Cholesterol 106mg

○ Sodium 292mg

○ Carbohydrate 7g
Fiber 1g

○ Protein 29g

PREPARATION TIP
Try using Rock Cornish hen instead of chicken. It has a pleasant, mild, gamey flavor.

Preparation Time: 50 minutes, plus 30 minutes marinating
Serves: 4

ORIENTAL GINGER CHICKEN

THE AROMATIC GARLIC, GINGER, AND SESAME OIL

MARINADE ADDS A CHINESE FLAVOR TO THIS SIMPLE MAIN

COURSE DISH. SERVE IT WITH PLAIN RICE OR NOODLES

AND A MIXED GREEN SALAD.

*4 skinless chicken breast halves, each about 4oz (125g),
sliced into ½in (1cm) strips*
*4 scallions, finely shredded, green parts
removed and reserved*
1 carrot, sliced into fine strips
*3 cups (100g) shiitake mushrooms, stems discarded,
and caps thinly sliced*
*1 cup (100g) thin asparagus tips or snow peas
freshly ground black pepper, to taste*

FOR THE MARINADE
1–2 hot chilies, seeded and finely chopped
1 clove garlic, finely chopped
1in (2.5cm) piece of fresh ginger, grated
1 tbsp reduced-salt soy sauce
1 tbsp dark brown sugar or honey
1 tbsp toasted sesame oil

1 Combine the marinade ingredients. Place the chicken in a shallow dish, then add the marinade. Turn the chicken in the marinade, rubbing it into the meat. Cover, and refrigerate for 30 minutes.

2 Place the chicken on a plate in a steamer. Spoon the marinade over the chicken. Arrange the vegetables, except the asparagus, over the chicken, and steam for 15–20 minutes, until the meat is tender.

3 Add the asparagus 5 minutes before the end of the cooking time, and cook, until just tender. Season, and garnish the chicken and vegetables with the reserved green parts of the scallions.

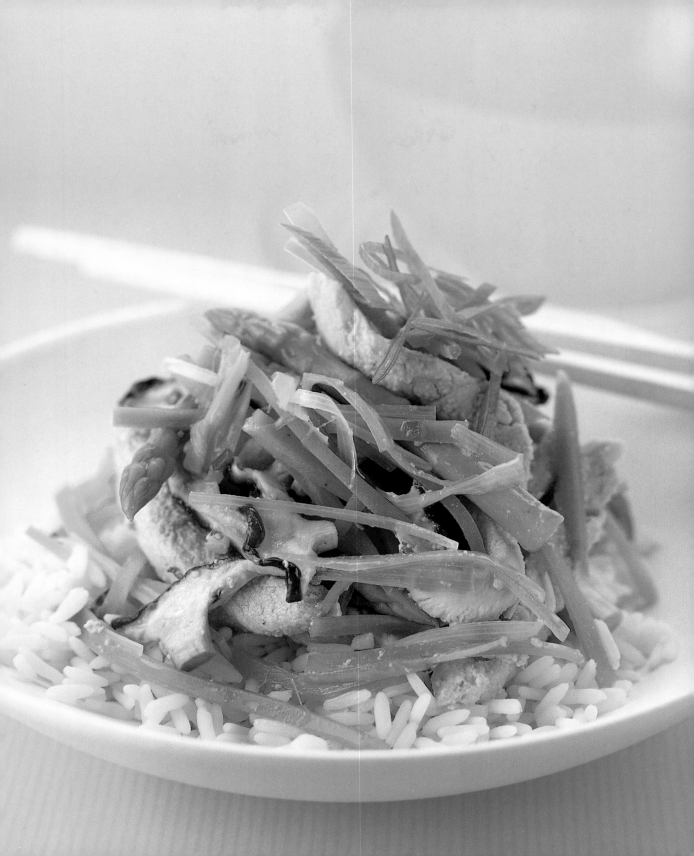

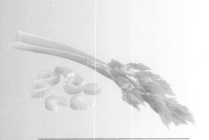

★ STAR INGREDIENT
Celery contains fiber and a
range of vitamins and minerals
that all contribute to good health.

EACH SERVING PROVIDES:

- ○ Calories 240

- ○ Total Fat 6g
  Saturated Fat 2g
  Polyunsaturated Fat 2g
  Monounsaturated Fat 2g

- ○ Cholesterol 74mg

- ○ Sodium 160mg

- ○ Carbohydrate 25g
  Fiber 4g

- ○ Protein 24g

PREPARATION TIP
The flavor of this dish improves
if kept overnight in the
refrigerator. Store covered,
removing from the refrigerator
an hour before serving.

Preparation Time: 55 minutes,
plus 1 hour chilling
Serves: 4

Turkey Meatballs

HERBED TURKEY MEATBALLS ARE BAKED IN A RICH,

SPICY TOMATO SAUCE. THE MEATBALLS CAN BE SERVED OVER

STEAMED BROWN RICE OR PASTA WITH MARINATED & BROILED

MUSHROOMS (*SEE PAGE 97*) AND A SALAD.

1 small onion, chopped
3 celery sticks, with their green leaves, chopped
1 small hot chili, seeded and chopped
small bunch of fresh parsley, stalks removed
1–2 sprigs of thyme, leaves finely chopped
11½oz (350g) ground turkey breast
½ cup (75g) cooked pearl barley
1 egg white
3–4 tbsp dried breadcrumbs or matzo meal
salt and freshly ground black pepper, to taste
1 quantity Spicy Tomato Sauce (see page 120)

1 Place the onion, celery, chili, and parsley in a food processor, and mix until finely chopped but not puréed.

2 Transfer the mixture to a bowl, then add the thyme, chicken, barley, egg white, breadcrumbs, and seasoning, and mix well. Cover, and refrigerate for about 1 hour.

3 Preheat the oven to 400°F (200°C). Cover the bottom of a baking dish with half the tomato sauce, then place rounded tablespoonfuls of the chicken mixture on top. Cover with the remaining sauce, and bake, uncovered, basting the chicken balls occasionally, for 30–45 minutes, until they are cooked and tender.

VARIATION
Chicken Meatballs Ground chicken can be substituted for the turkey, although it is more difficult to find and higher in fat than turkey.

CHICKEN CASSEROLE

THIS SATISFYING, HEARTY DISH IS A PERFECT "COMFORT FOOD"

FOR COLD WINTER EVENINGS. THE NUTRITIOUS COMBINATION

OF HIGH-FIBER BEANS, GARLIC, VEGETABLES, AND CHICKEN

MAKES A COMPLETE MEAL IN ITSELF.

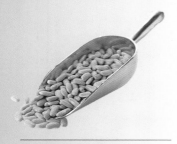

✴ STAR INGREDIENT
Flageolet beans, like other beans, are a good source of soluble fiber, which may lower blood-cholesterol levels.

EACH SERVING PROVIDES:

○ Calories 346

○ Total Fat 10g
　Saturated Fat 2g
　Polyunsaturated Fat 2g
　Monounsaturated Fat 6g

○ Cholesterol 64mg

○ Sodium 211mg

○ Carbohydrate 32g
　Fiber 10g

○ Protein 33g

SERVING TIP
This dish can be served on its own or over rice, bulgar, or couscous, and with a steamed green vegetable.

PREPARATION TIP
Add extra stock or water to the casserole in step 4 if it appears too dry.

Preparation Time: 1 hour, 20 minutes
Serves: 4

1½ tbsp olive oil
6 skinless, boneless chicken thighs, each about 3oz (75g),
cut into bite-sized pieces
1 large onion, finely chopped
4 cloves garlic, coarsely chopped
1 large carrot, coarsely chopped
5 tbsp water
2 cups (150g) cremini mushrooms, sliced
½ cups (15g) dried porcini mushrooms, rehydrated in hot water
for 20 minutes (optional)
3 tbsp chopped fresh thyme, or ¼ tsp dried thyme
1 cup (200g) dried flageolet or lima beans, cooked, or
13oz (400g) canned beans in water (rinsed)
1¼–1½ cups (300–400ml) hot chicken or vegetable stock
(see pages 118–19)
freshly ground black pepper, to taste

1 Preheat the oven to 400°F (200°C). Heat the oil in a large, heavy-based saucepan. Add the chicken pieces and cook over a medium heat for 3–4 minutes, until browned all over, then set aside. Add the onion, garlic, and carrot to the pan, and cook for a further 1–2 minutes.

2 Add the water to the pan, and cook the vegetables over a medium heat for 5–6 minutes, stirring occasionally, until the water evaporates and the onion starts to brown. Remove the pan from the heat, then stir in the browned chicken and all the mushrooms.

3 Spoon a layer of the chicken and vegetables into an ovenproof casserole. Sprinkle with a third of the thyme and a third of the beans. Continue to layer until all the ingredients have been used.

4 Pour the stock over the layered ingredients and season. Cover, and bake for 45 minutes, stirring occasionally. Uncover, and bake for a further 10–15 minutes, until the chicken is tender.

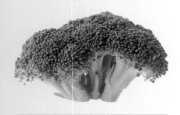

✱ STAR INGREDIENT
Broccoli is rich in many vitamins and minerals, particularly the antioxidants vitamin C and beta-carotene, as well as folate, which are all thought to protect against heart disease.

EACH SERVING PROVIDES:

○ Calories 460

○ Total Fat 10g
  Saturated Fat 2g
  Polyunsaturated Fat 4g
  Monounsaturated Fat 3g

○ Cholesterol 88mg

○ Sodium mg

○ Carbohydrate 54g
  Fiber 1g

○ Protein 38g

PREPARATION TIP
Skinless chicken breast is low in fat and consequently can dry out during cooking. To retain a moist texture, cook it quickly until tender.

1 lb of sea scallops or shrimp, both very low in fat, can be used instead of chicken.

Preparation Time: 40 minutes
Serves: 4

CHICKEN NOODLE STIR-FRY

STIR-FRYING IS A CLASSIC LOW FAT COOKING METHOD, AND IS INCREDIBLY VERSATILE. THIS SIMPLE DISH INCLUDES A HEALTHY COMBINATION OF GARLIC, CHILIES, SHIITAKE MUSHROOMS, AND BROCCOLI, ALL GOOD FOR THE HEART.

1 tbsp sunflower or light olive oil
½ tbsp toasted sesame oil
*4 skinless chicken breast halves, each about 4oz (125g),
sliced into ½in (1cm) strips*
5 tbsp water
4–5 cloves garlic, thinly sliced
2–3 mild red chilies, seeded and cut into fine strips
1 bunch scallions, chopped, the green parts reserved to garnish
*2 cups (150g) shiitake mushrooms, stems discarded,
and caps thickly sliced*
1 tbsp reduced-salt soy sauce
1¼ cups (300ml) chicken stock (see page 119)
1 tsp cornstarch, mixed with 1 tbsp white wine
2 cups (150g) broccoli florets, lightly steamed
*2 cups (250g) dried thin rice noodles, soaked
in boiling water for 3 minutes*

1 Heat the sunflower and sesame oils in a large wok or frying pan. Add the chicken, and stir-fry over a high heat for 4–5 minutes, until the meat has browned. Remove the meat from the wok and keep warm.

2 Reduce the heat to medium. Add the water and mix it with the wok juices. Add the garlic, chilies, and scallions, reserving the green parts. Stir-fry for a further 3–4 minutes, until the onions start to soften.

3 Add the shiitake mushrooms and the soy sauce, and stir-fry for 2–3 minutes, until they have softened. Add the stock and bring the mixture to a boil. Reduce the heat, then simmer gently for 15 minutes, or until the stock has slightly reduced.

4 Increase the heat, stir in the cornstarch mixture, and bring to a boil. Add the chicken, broccoli, and noodles. Cook for 5–6 minutes, until all the ingredients are heated through and the chicken is tender. Garnish with the green parts of the scallions before serving.

FILET MIGNON WITH THREE-PEPPER SALSA

LEANER AND CONSEQUENTLY LOWER IN FAT THAN MOST OTHER RED MEATS, FILET MIGNON IS AN EXCELLENT CHOICE FOR MEAT LOVERS. SERVE WITH ORIENTAL MUSHROOM RISOTTO (*SEE PAGE 55*).

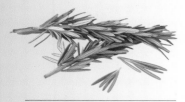

★ STAR INGREDIENT
Due to its high essential oil content, fresh rosemary is thought to benefit the nervous system.

EACH SERVING PROVIDES:

○ Calories 300

○ Total Fat 11g
Saturated Fat 2g
Polyunsaturated Fat 4g
Monounsaturated Fat 5g

○ Cholesterol 88mg

○ Sodium 103mg

○ Carbohydrate 9g
Fiber 3g

○ Protein 41g

SERVING TIP
Serve the filet mignon with a green salad or steamed or broiled vegetables.

Preparation Time: 35 minutes, plus 1 hour chilling
Serves: 4

1 tbsp olive oil
2 cloves garlic, crushed
juice of ½ lemon
1 tbsp mustard
1 tbsp chopped fresh rosemary
4 filet mignon steaks, each about 4oz (125g)

FOR THE SALSA
1 large red pepper, halved, cored, and seeded
1 large yellow or orange pepper, halved, cored, and seeded
1 large green pepper, halved, cored, and seeded
1 tbsp sunflower oil
1 small red onion, finely chopped
1 clove garlic, crushed
1–2 chilies, seeded and finely chopped (optional)
2 tbsp wine vinegar
2 tbsp chopped fresh thyme
freshly ground black pepper, to taste

1 Mix together the oil, garlic, lemon juice, mustard, and rosemary to form a thick paste. Spread the paste evenly over both sides of each steak. Cover, and refrigerate for about 1 hour.

2 Preheat the broiler. Lightly brush the peppers with the oil, and broil for 5–7 minutes, until charred and blistered. Transfer the peppers to a plastic bag and seal. Leave the peppers for 5 minutes, then peel under cold, running water and finely chop.

3 Place the peppers and the rest of the salsa ingredients in a bowl. Cover, and refrigerate for 30 minutes. Preheat the broiler to high. Broil the steaks for 5–6 minutes on each side, or until cooked according to preference. Serve with the salsa.

Venison Burgers

THESE JUICY BURGERS ARE EASY TO MAKE AND LOW IN FAT.

ADDING A MINCED CLOVE OF GARLIC IN THE BURGER MIXTURE

GIVES A WONDERFUL TASTE AND AROMA. SERVE IN A BUN WITH

CARAMELIZED ONION & POTATO SALAD (SEE PAGE 91).

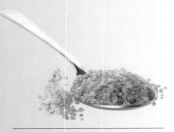

✱ STAR INGREDIENT
Bulgar wheat is low in sodium and high in carbohydrate, making it a useful staple in a healthy heart diet.

EACH SERVING PROVIDES:

○ Calories 190

○ Total Fat 6g
  Saturated Fat 1g
  Polyunsaturated Fat 3g
  Monounsaturated Fat 1g

○ Cholesterol 44mg

○ Sodium 83mg

○ Carbohydrate 14g
  Fiber 2g

○ Protein 22g

PREPARATION TIP
Try adding different vegetables, such as finely chopped zucchini, or mushrooms to these burgers, or even fruits like apples and pears.

Preparation Time: 30 minutes, plus 1 hour chilling
Serves: 4

11½oz (350g) ground venison
1 onion, finely chopped
2 celery sticks, finely chopped
1 small carrot, finely grated
¼ cup (50g) bulgar, soaked in hot water for 30 minutes, drained, and squeezed dry
4 tbsp chopped fresh flat-leaf parsley, stalks removed
1 egg white
salt and freshly ground black pepper, to taste
1 tbsp sunflower oil

To Garnish
2 shallots or onions, thinly sliced
4 sprigs of redcurrants
lettuce and sliced tomatos

1 Place all the ingredients, except the oil and garnishes, in a large bowl and mix well until thoroughly combined. (This can alternatively be done in a food processor with either the beater or the dough-hook attachment.) Cover, and refrigerate for about 1 hour.

2 Preheat the broiler. Divide the mixture into 4 equal portions, then shape each one into a burger about 1in (2.5cm) thick. Lightly brush with the oil, then broil for 5–8 minutes on each side, until browned. (Alternatively, cook them for the same length of time in a non-stick frying pan.) Garnish with the shallots, sprigs of redcurrants, lettuce, and sliced tomato.

VARIATION
Chicken Burgers Replace the venison with 11½oz (350g) ground chicken or turkey breast. Increase the quantity of bulgar to ½ cup (75g) and flavor the mixture with 1–2 red chilies, seeded and finely chopped. Replace the parsley with 4 tablespoons of chopped cilantro.

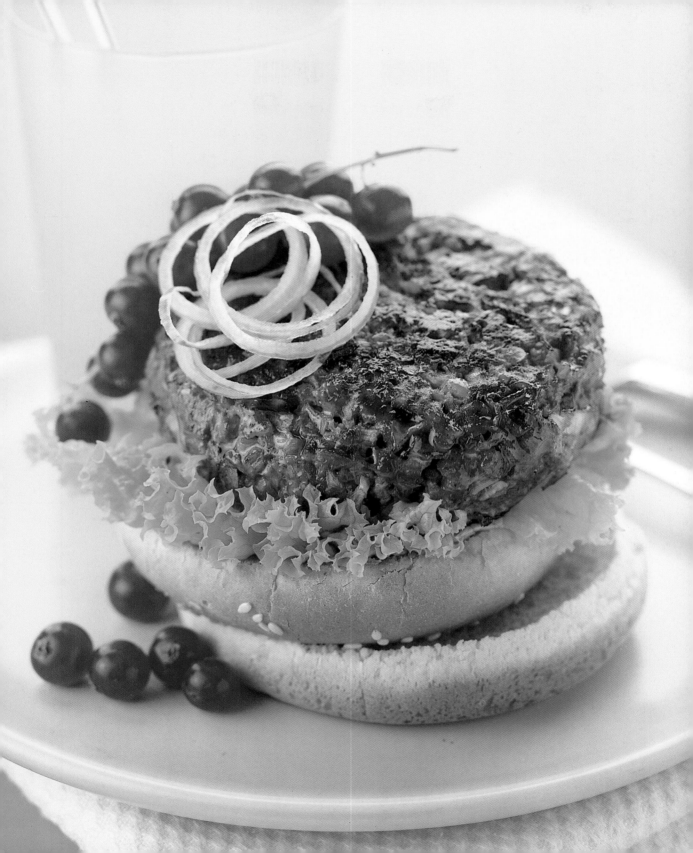

HEARTY PORK STEW

PORK LOIN IS MARKETED AS THE "OTHER WHITE MEAT" BECAUSE IT IS

VERY LOW IN FAT AND CHOLESTEROL. SERVE THIS RICH STEW WITH

RICE OR PASTA, OR WITH WHOLEWHEAT CROUTONS.

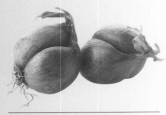

★ STAR INGREDIENT
Shallots contain sulfur compounds that may help to control cholesterol levels, as well as quercetin, which may protect against heart disease.

EACH SERVING PROVIDES:

○ Calories 280

○ Total Fat 10g
　Saturated Fat 3g
　Polyunsaturated Fat 3g
　Monounsaturated Fat 4g

○ Cholesterol 66mg

○ Sodium 159mg

○ Carbohydrate 16g
　Fiber 2g

○ Protein 32g

PREPARATION TIP
Alternatively, this recipe can be made with rabbit, chicken, turkey, or veal.

Preparation Time: 1 hour, 15 minutes, plus 30 minutes marinating
Serves: 4

2 tbsp lemon juice
grated peel of ½ orange
1 tbsp olive oil
1lb (500g) pork loin, trimmed of fat and cut into bite-sized pieces
6 small shallots, quartered
6 large cloves garlic, quartered
3 celery sticks, finely chopped
juice of 2 oranges
1¼ cups (300ml) chicken or vegetable stock (see pages 118–19)
bouquet garni, made up of 3 sprigs of thyme,
2 sprigs of rosemary, and 1 bay leaf
freshly ground black pepper, to taste
½ cup (100g) ready-to-eat dried prunes
fresh thyme, to garnish

1 Combine the lemon juice, grated orange peel, and half the oil, then pour the mixture over the rabbit in a shallow dish. Turn the meat in the marinade. Cover, and refrigerate for 30 minutes.

2 Heat a heavy-based saucepan over a low heat and sauté the pork loin for 8 minutes, turning occasionally, until browned. Set aside, and keep warm. Heat the remaining oil in the pan. Add the shallots, garlic, and celery, and saute for 5 minutes, or until browned. Add the orange juice, stock, bouquet garni, and seasoning. Bring to a boil, then reduce the heat and simmer for 2 minutes. Add the pork loin and bring to a rapid boil, turning the pork pieces in the boiling liquid, then season.

3 Reduce the heat and add the prunes. Cover, and simmer, skimming away any froth, for 45 minutes, or until the pork is tender. Remove the pork, and keep hot. Remove and discard the bouquet garni, then return the liquid to a boil, and boil hard for 8–10 minutes, until the liquid has reduced by half. Return the meat to the pan and heat through. Garnish with the thyme before serving.

FRUITY VEGETABLE CURRY

THIS AROMATIC BLEND OF GARLIC, GINGER, CINNAMON, AND STOCK
MAKES A RICH SAUCE FOR BABY VEGETABLES AND APPLES. BASED ON A
CLASSIC RECIPE, THIS CURRY IS BEST SERVED WITH RICE AND TOPPED
WITH A SPOONFUL OF FAT-FREE PLAIN YOGURT.

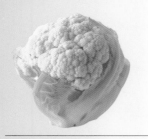

✴ STAR INGREDIENT
Cauliflower is a cruciferous
vegetable and is full of valuable
nutrients, including potassium,
fiber, vitamins C and E, folate,
and beta-carotene.

EACH SERVING PROVIDES:

○ Calories 130

○ Total Fat 6g
  Saturated Fat 1g
  Polyunsaturated Fat 2g
  Monounsaturated Fat 3g

○ Cholesterol 0mg

○ Sodium 111mg

○ Carbohydrate 18g
  Fiber 4g

○ Protein 5g

Preparation Time: 35 minutes
Serves: 4

1 onion, finely chopped
4 cloves garlic, chopped
1in (2.5cm) piece of fresh ginger, chopped
1 carrot, coarsely chopped
1 tbsp peanut oil
1 tbsp mustard seeds
2 red chilies, seeded and chopped
4 cardamom pods
1 small cinnamon stick
½ tsp turmeric
4 tbsp cider or white wine vinegar
2 apples, peeled, cored, and coarsely chopped
1¾ cups (400ml) hot vegetable stock (see page 118), or water
1 tbsp honey or brown sugar
freshly ground black pepper, to taste
13oz (400g) baby vegetables, such as cauliflower,
broccoli, or cabbage, quartered and lightly steamed
2 tbsp fresh cilantro, to garnish

1 In a food processor, blend together the onion, garlic, ginger, and
carrot into a thick paste.

2 Heat the oil in a heavy-based saucepan. Add the mustard seeds,
chilies, and spices. Cook over a medium heat until the mustard seeds
start to pop and emit a pleasant, toasted aroma. Add the onion/carrot
paste and cook over a high heat, stirring frequently, for 5–6 minutes,
until the mixture starts to color. Add 3–4 tablespoons of water if the
mixture becomes too dry.

3 Add the vinegar, apples, stock, honey, and seasoning. Bring to a
boil, then reduce the heat. Simmer, uncovered, for 10 minutes, or until
the apples are tender. Add the vegetables and simmer for 4–5 minutes
to heat through. Garnish with the cilantro before serving.

Artichoke & Fava Bean Stew

THIS LIGHT, YET SATISFYING SUMMER STEW CONTAINS A HEALTHY

COMBINATION OF HIGH-FIBER FAVA BEANS AND VITAMIN-RICH

VEGETABLES. SERVE IT WITH MULTIGRAIN BREAD OR RICE.

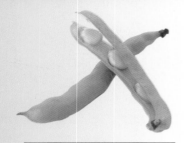

✴ STAR INGREDIENT

Fava beans are a good source of beta-carotene and soluble fiber and also contain some iron and vitamins C and E.

EACH SERVING PROVIDES:

○ Calories 181

○ Total Fat 5g
   Saturated Fat 1g
   Polyunsaturated Fat 1g
   Monounsaturated Fat 3g

○ Cholesterol 0mg

○ Sodium 145mg

○ Carbohydrate 24g
   Fiber 11g

○ Protein 13g

PREPARATION TIP

Chicken stock can be used instead of the vegetable stock, if preferred.

Preparation Time: 1 hour, 10 minutes
Serves: 4

1 tbsp olive oil
1 bunch of scallions, shredded
4–5 cloves garlic, coarsely chopped
2 large carrots, chopped
2 celery sticks, finely chopped
2 cups (500ml) vegetable stock (see pages 118–19)
bouquet garni, made with 2–3 sprigs of thyme,
1–2 sprigs of rosemary, and 2 strips of lemon peel
13oz (400g) canned artichoke hearts, drained and quartered
2½ cups (400g) fava beans or canned chickpeas in water
juice of 1 lemon, mixed with 1 tsp sugar
freshly ground black pepper, to taste
sprigs of fresh thyme, to garnish

1 Heat the oil in a heavy-based saucepan. Add the scallions, garlic, carrots, and celery. Sauté over a medium heat for 5–8 minutes, until the vegetables have softened. Add the stock and bouquet garni, then bring to a boil. Cook for 4–5 minutes, until the liquid has reduced.

2 Reduce the heat, then add the artichoke hearts and fava beans to the pan. Simmer, half-covered, for 30–45 minutes, until most of the liquid has evaporated. Stir in the lemon juice mixture. Season, and garnish with the thyme before serving.

Variation

Stew with Added Chicken Slice 4 x 4oz (125g) skinless chicken breast halves into ½in (1cm) strips. Cook them on a dry skillet or non-stick frying pan for 3–4 minutes on each side, until browned. Add the chicken to the stew 10 minutes before the end of the cooking time.

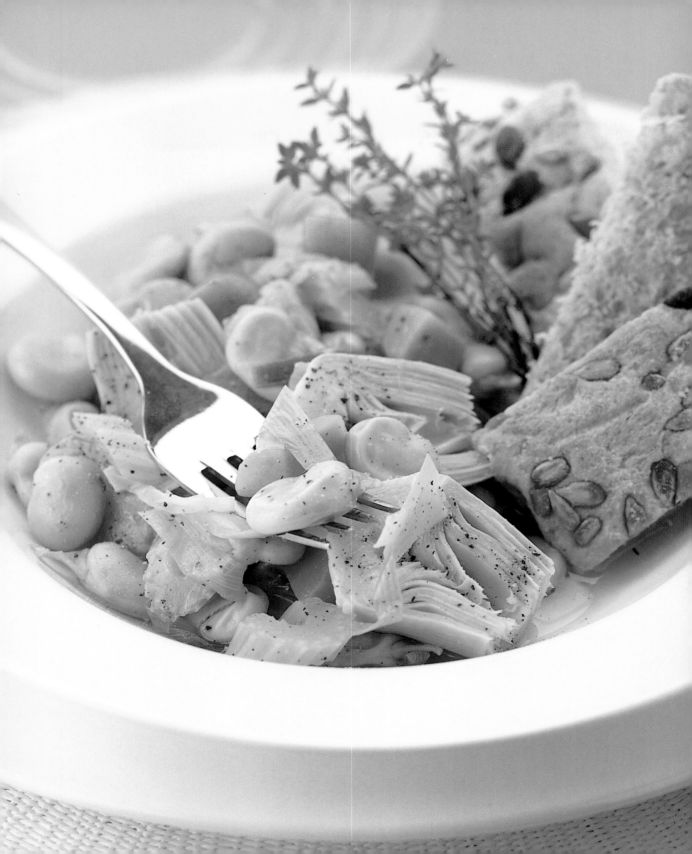

CHINESE MIXED MUSHROOM STEW

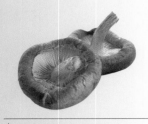

IN ASIA, EATING ORIENTAL MUSHROOMS IS RECOMMENDED FOR A

LONG AND HEALTHY LIFE. THEY ARE USED IN ABUNDANCE IN THIS DISH,

WHICH IS DELICIOUS SERVED WITH RICE, NOODLES, OR BULGAR.

2 tbsp peanut or sesame oil
7 large (100g) shallots, quartered
4 cloves garlic, thickly sliced
1–2 mild chilies, seeded and finely chopped (optional)
1½ cups (125g) oyster mushrooms, broken into chunks
1¼ cups (100g) shiitake mushrooms, or 1 cup (50g) dried shiitake,
rehydrated in hot water for 20 minutes, stems discarded,
and caps sliced
1 tbsp reduced-salt soy sauce
1¾ cups (400ml) vegetable or chicken stock (see pages 118–19)
2 cups (250g) dried thin rice noodles,
soaked in boiling water for 3 minutes
2 tbsp chopped fresh dill, to garnish

1 Heat the oil in a wok or heavy-based frying pan. Add the shallots, garlic, and chilies, if using, and stir-fry over a high heat for 3–4 minutes, until they start to brown. Add the oyster and shiitake mushrooms and stir-fry for a further 4–5 minutes, until the mushrooms have softened. Add the soy sauce and stir-fry for 1–2 minutes.

2 Add the stock, and bring to a boil. Reduce the heat and simmer for 15 minutes, until the stock has reduced.

3 Increase the heat to medium, add the noodles and cook, folding the noodles into the mushroom sauce, until almost all the liquid has evaporated and the noodles are glossy. Garnish with the dill.

✷ STAR INGREDIENT
Studies have found that oriental mushrooms, including shiitake and oyster, may help to lower blood-cholesterol levels, even possibly reducing the effects of saturated fat in the body.

EACH SERVING PROVIDES:

○ Calories 360

○ Total Fat 8g
   Saturated Fat 2g
   Polyunsaturated Fat 2g
   Monounsaturated Fat 3g

○ Cholesterol 0mg

○ Sodium 285mg

○ Carbohydrate 60g
   Fiber 1g

○ Protein 9g

PREPARATION TIP
Use portabello or cremini mushrooms instead of oyster mushrooms, if desired.

Preparation Time: 40 minutes
Serves: 4

MIXED GRAIN CASSEROLE

SERVE THIS WARM AND SATISFYING WINTER DISH WITH WHOLEWHEAT

BREAD AND A GLASS OF FULL-BODIED RED WINE.

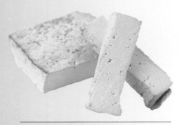

✳ STAR INGREDIENT
Tofu is low in fat and rich in potassium, calcium, and isoflavins, which may reduce the risk of heart disease.

EACH SERVING PROVIDES:

○ Calories 340

○ Total Fat 9g
  Saturated Fat 1g
  Polyunsaturated Fat 2g
  Monounsaturated Fat 5g

○ Cholesterol 0mg

○ Sodium 309mg

○ Carbohydrate 52g
  Fiber 7g

○ Protein 14g

PREPARATION TIPS
You can prepare the casserole in advance and store it covered in the refrigerator for up to 2 days. Wheat berries are the whole wheat grain and are readily available from health food shops.

Preparation Time: 2 hours, 25 minutes, plus soaking overnight
Serves: 4

⅓ cup (60g) wheat berries, soaked overnight
⅓ cup (60g) millet, soaked overnight
⅓ cup (60g) pearl barley, soaked overnight
1½ tbsp olive oil
1 large onion, coarsely chopped
3 carrots, coarsely chopped
2–3 celery sticks, coarsely chopped
¾ cup (50g) dried shiitake mushrooms, rehydrated in
½ cup (100ml) boiling water for 30 minutes, stems discarded,
and caps thickly sliced, and the soaking water reserved
5oz (150g) firm tofu, cubed
bouquet garni, made up of 3–4 sprigs of thyme,
1–2 sprigs of marjoram, and 2 strips of lemon peel
1 tsp caraway seeds
freshly ground black pepper, to taste
2 cups (500ml) chicken or vegetable stock
(see pages 118–19)
1 tbsp reduced-salt soy sauce

1 Preheat the oven to 400°F (200°C). Drain the wheat berries, millet, and pearl barley, and mix together. Heat the oil in a large frying pan, and add the onion, carrots, and celery. Sauté over a medium heat for 5–8 minutes, until the onion starts to brown. Stir in the mushrooms and cook for a further 3 minutes.

2 Arrange a third of the grains in the bottom of a large casserole, and top with a third of the vegetable mixture and half of the tofu. Cover with another layer of grains, vegetables, and the rest of the tofu. Top with a final layer of grains and vegetables.

3 Place the bouquet garni over the grains and vegetables. Scatter the caraway seeds over the top and season. Pour in the stock, soy sauce, and reserved mushroom water. Cover, and bake for 1½–2 hours, until the grains are tender. Check the casserole ocassionally, adding extra water if it becomes too dry.

Roasted Red Pepper & Chickpea Salad

SWEET RED PEPPERS COMPLEMENT THE NUTTY FLAVOR OF THE
CHICKPEAS IN THIS SIMPLE, COLORFUL SALAD. IT MAKES A
DELICIOUS ACCOMPANIMENT TO BROILED CHICKEN OR FISH.

2 x 15oz (850g) cans chickpeas, drained and rinsed
4 red peppers, cored, seeded, and quartered

For the Dressing
1 tbsp balsamic vinegar
2 tbsp extra-virgin olive oil
4 scallions, finely chopped
1 clove garlic, finely chopped
2 tbsp chopped mixed fresh herbs,
such as parsley, thyme, and sage
freshly ground black pepper, to taste

1 Mix together the dressing ingredients in a large bowl.

2 Preheat the broiler. Brush the skins of the peppers with a little of the dressing, then broil for 8–10 minutes, until the skins have blistered and blackened. Place the peppers in a plastic bag and leave for 5 minutes, then peel and slice.

3 Stir the peppers into the dressing, then add the chickpeas, and mix well. Allow to cool before serving.

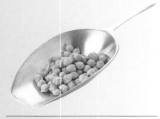

★ STAR INGREDIENT
Chickpeas are a low fat source of protein and rich in soluble fiber, which may help to lower blood cholesterol levels.

EACH SERVING PROVIDES:

○ Calories 195

○ Total Fat 10g
  Saturated Fat 1g
  Polyunsaturated Fat 2g
  Monounsaturated Fat 6g

○ Cholesterol 0mg

○ Sodium 19mg

○ Carbohydrate 21g
  Fiber 5g

○ Protein 7g

BUYING TIP
Canned beans are an excellent and convenient alternative to dried. Buy them in water, rather than in brine, without salt and sugar, and drain well.

Preparation Time: 30 minutes
Serves: 4

SALADS *Fresh and nutritious, these*
mouthwatering salads can be served as appetizers, accompaniments, or light
main meals. If you go easy on salad dressings, these dishes are impressive
low sodium and low fat sources of vitamins, minerals and fiber.

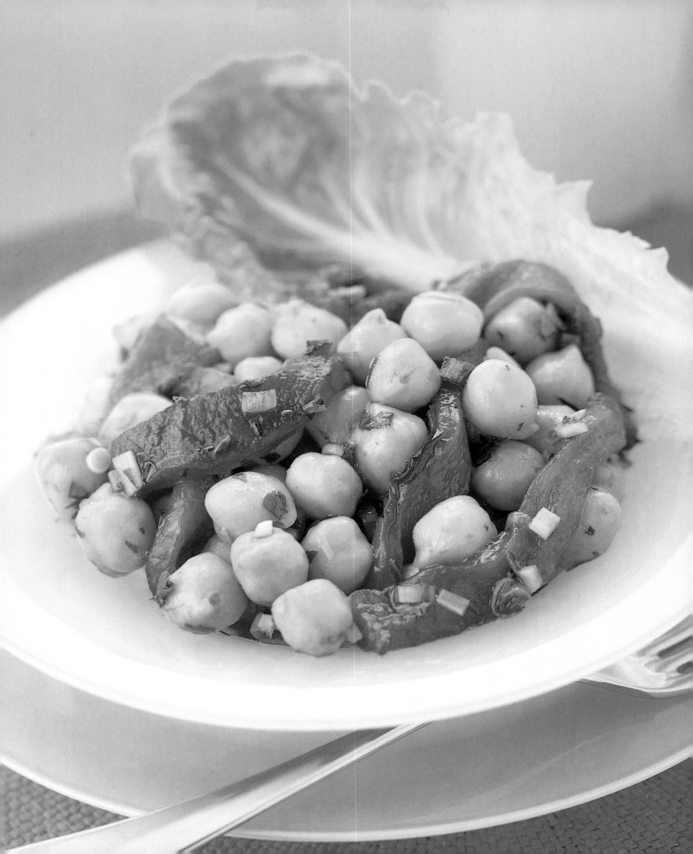

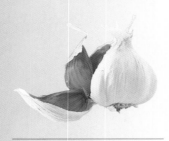

ROASTED GARLIC & ZUCCHINI SALAD

GARLIC IS AN IMPORTANT INGREDIENT IN THE HEALTHY HEART

KITCHEN. IT LOSES ITS PUNGENCY WHEN ROASTED, BECOMING SOFT,

CREAMY, AND DELICIOUS.

12–16 large cloves garlic, peeled and quartered
juice of 1 orange and 1 tsp grated peel
1 tbsp olive oil
2–3 cloves (optional)
1–2 tsp brown sugar
6 zucchini, sliced with a potato peeler into ribbons
freshly ground black pepper, to taste
1 tbsp chopped fresh dill or lemon thyme

1 Preheat the oven to 400°F (200°C). Place the garlic in a baking dish, then spoon over 3 tablespoons of the orange juice and the grated peel, oil, cloves, if using, and sugar. Cover with foil, and bake for 15–20 minutes, until the garlic starts to soften.

2 Pour boiling water over the zucchini and blanch for a few seconds until slightly softened. Drain well and pat dry with a kitchen towel, getting rid of as much moisture as possible.

3 Increase the oven setting to 450°F (230°C). Uncover the baking dish, then stir in the zucchini, and the remaining orange juice. Bake for a further 10–15 minutes, until the garlic and zucchini start to caramelize. Season, and sprinkle with the fresh herbs. Serve either hot or at room temperature.

✳ STAR INGREDIENT
The benefits of garlic are wide-ranging. It has been shown to improve the circulation, and reduce both blood pressure and blood cholesterol levels.

EACH SERVING PROVIDES:

○ Calories 80

○ Total Fat 4g
 Saturated Fat <1g
 Polyunsaturated Fat <1g
 Monounsaturated Fat 3g

○ Cholesterol 0mg

○ Sodium 3mg

○ Carbohydrate 7g
 Fiber 2g

○ Protein 3g

SERVING TIP
When roasted, garlic makes a wonderfully creamy, low-fat sandwich spread.

Preparation Time: 45 minutes
Serves: 4

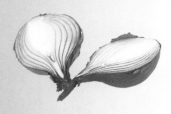

CARAMELIZED ONION & POTATO SALAD

THE CARAMELIZED ONIONS LEND A DELICIOUS SWEETNESS TO THE

WARM NEW POTATOES. AS AN ADDED BONUS, POTATOES PROVIDE

ENERGY AS WELL AS FIBER AND VITAMIN C.

1lb (500g) small salad potatoes
2 large onions, thinly sliced
4 tbsp water
2 tbsp olive or sunflower oil
6 tbsp balsamic vinegar
freshly ground black pepper, to taste
1 tsp caraway seeds, roasted in a dry frying pan,
and crushed
4 tbsp chopped, fresh flat-leaf parsley or mint

1 Steam the potatoes for 15 minutes, or until tender, then keep hot.

2 Meanwhile, put the onions and water in a small saucepan and bring to a boil. Reduce the heat, cover, and simmer for 10 minutes, or until the onions are tender and the water has evaporated.

3 Add the oil to the saucepan, and cook, stirring constantly, for a further 5 minutes, or until the onions start to caramelize. Add the vinegar and bring to a boil. Cook for 1–2 minutes, until the liquid has reduced and is glossy.

4 Pour the onion mixture over the hot potatoes in a large bowl, and mix well. Cover the bowl with a clean cloth and let the potatoes cool to room temperature. Season to taste, and sprinkle with the caraway seeds and flat-leaf parsley before serving.

✳ STAR INGREDIENT

Onions, like garlic, contain allicin compounds that help to fight infections and lower cholesterol levels, as well as protecting against cancer.

EACH SERVING PROVIDES:

○ Calories 190

○ Total Fat 8g
   Saturated Fat 1g
   Polyunsaturated Fat 1g
   Monounsaturated Fat 6g

○ Cholesterol 0mg

○ Sodium 15mg

○ Carbohydrate 27g
   Fiber 3g

○ Protein 4g

PREPARATION TIP

Do not peel the potatoes – wash and scrub them instead to retain their fiber and vitamin content.

Preparation Time: 25 minutes, plus 5 minutes cooling
Serves: 4

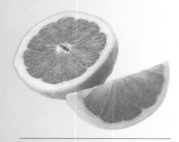

FENNEL & RUBY GRAPEFRUIT SALAD

THIS REFRESHING SALAD IS EXCELLENT WITH GRILLED FISH OR CHICKEN.

LIKE OTHER CITRUS FRUITS, GRAPEFRUIT CONTAINS HIGH AMOUNTS

OF VITAMIN C, WHILE FENNEL IS A WELL-KNOWN DIURETIC.

2 large fennel bulbs, cored and thinly sliced,
leafy tops reserved, to garnish
2 large ruby grapefruit, segmented
1 small red or white onion, thinly sliced into rings
1 red chili, seeded and finely chopped
1 tbsp hazelnut oil
2 tsp clear honey
2 tbsp chopped fresh dill
freshly ground black pepper, to taste

Combine the fennel (reserving the leafy tops to garnish) and grapefruit in a large serving bowl. Add the rest of the ingredients, then mix well until combined. Garnish with the reserved fennel leafy tops.

VARIATION
Orange and Chicory Salad Replace the fennel and grapefruit with 3 oranges, segmented, and 3 heads of chicory, thinly sliced.

★ STAR INGREDIENT
Grapefruit contains high amounts of pectin, which has been found to lower blood cholesterol levels.

EACH SERVING PROVIDES:

○ Calories 120

○ Total Fat 4g
   Saturated Fat <1g
   Polyunsaturated Fat <1g
   Monounsaturated Fat 3g

○ Cholesterol 0mg

○ Sodium 28mg

○ Carbohydrate 17g
   Fiber 7g

○ Protein 3g

Preparation Time: 15 minutes
Serves: 4

EACH SERVING PROVIDES:

- ○ Calories 110
- ○ Total Fat 4g
  - Saturated Fat <1g
  - Polyunsaturated Fat <1g
  - Monounsaturated Fat 3g
- ○ Cholesterol 0mg
- ○ Sodium 113mg
- ○ Carbohydrate 16g
  - Fiber 3g
- ○ Protein 2g

Preparation Time: 15 minutes, plus 1 hour chilling
Serves: 4

BEET SALAD WITH HONEY & YOGURT DRESSING

BEET IS ONE OF NATURE'S MOST EFFECTIVE DETOXIFIERS, HELPING

TO CLEANSE BOTH THE LIVER AND THE KIDNEYS. ITS NATURAL

SWEETNESS ENHANCES THE FLAVOR OF THE PINEAPPLE.

2 medium (300g) raw beets, coarsely grated
1 small pineapple, peeled, cored, and chopped
3 shallots or 1 small onion, finely chopped

FOR THE DRESSING
juice of 1 lemon
2 tbsp honey mustard
3 tbsp fat-free plain yogurt
1 tbsp olive or sunflower oil
freshly ground black pepper, to taste

Mix together the dressing ingredients, and pour over the beets, pineapple, and shallots. Refrigerate for about 1 hour before serving.

EACH SERVING PROVIDES:

- ○ Calories 100
- ○ Total Fat 4g
  - Saturated Fat <1g
  - Polyunsaturated Fat <1g
  - Monounsaturated Fat 3g
- ○ Cholesterol 0mg
- ○ Sodium 134mg
- ○ Carbohydrate 13g
  - Fiber 3g
- ○ Protein 2g

Preparation Time: 15 minutes, plus 1 hour standing
Serves: 4

CELERY & CARROT SALAD

1½ cups (200g) celery, finely grated
1½ cups (200g) carrots, finely grated

FOR THE DRESSING
juice of 1 orange and 1 tsp grated peel
juice of ½ lemon

2 tsp Dijon mustard
1 tbsp olive oil
2 tbsp golden raisins or raisins, soaked in a little orange juice for 20 minutes
freshly ground black pepper, to taste

Mix together the dressing ingredients, and pour over the celery and carrots. Refrigerate for about 1 hour before serving.

TUNA & BEAN SALAD

BASED ON AN ITALIAN CLASSIC, THIS SALAD IS A SUCCESSFUL
MARRIAGE OF LOW FAT, HIGH-FIBER BEANS, FRESH HERBS,
RED ONION, AND TUNA. SERVE IT AS A MAIN COURSE, IF DESIRED,
WITH WHOLEGRAIN BREAD.

7oz (200g) canned tuna chunks in spring water
1½ cups (220g) canned flageolet beans or lima beans, in water
1 red onion, sliced into paper-thin rings
1 clove garlic, crushed
1 Red Delicious apple, cored, and chopped
1 red pepper, cored, seeded, and finely chopped
4 tbsp chopped fresh flat-leaf parsley

FOR THE DRESSING
3 tbsp fat-free plain yogurt
*2 tsp honey mustard, or 1 tsp English mustard
mixed with 2 tsp honey*
1 tbsp extra-virgin olive oil
2 tbsp white wine vinegar, or lemon or lime juice
freshly ground black pepper, to taste

1 Mix together the dressing ingredients until combined.

2 Pour the dressing over the salad ingredients in a large serving bowl, and refrigerate for about 1 hour to allow the flavors to develop.

VARIATION
Chicken and Chickpea Salad Replace the tuna, beans, and apple with 10oz (300g) broiled, skinless, boneless chicken breast halves, 1½ cups (220g) canned chickpeas, and 1 pear, cored and chopped. Black beans can be used instead of the flageolet or lima beans as a delicious variation.

✻ STAR INGREDIENT
Tuna and other oily fish are rich in omega-3 fatty acids, which may help control cholesterol levels.

EACH SERVING PROVIDES:

○ Calories 170

○ Total Fat 5g
   Saturated Fat 1g
   Polyunsaturated Fat 1g
   Monounsaturated Fat 3g

○ Cholesterol 26mg

○ Sodium 330mg

○ Carbohydrate 15g
   Fiber 4g

○ Protein 17g

BUYING TIP
Try to avoid tuna packed in oil. Tuna in spring water has much lower levels of fat and can be rinsed to reduce the salt.

Preparation Time: 7 minutes, plus 1 hour chilling
Serves: 4

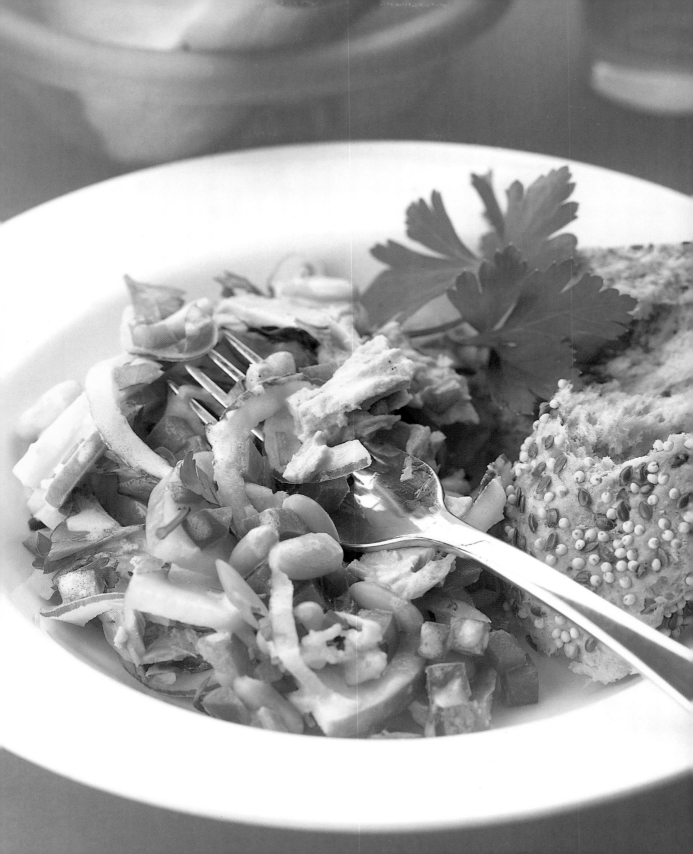

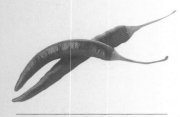

✳ STAR INGREDIENT
Chilies are a rich source of the antioxidant vitamin C, which helps neutralize cell damage caused by free radicals.

EACH SERVING PROVIDES:

○ Calories 110

○ Total Fat 8g
  Saturated Fat 1g
  Polyunsaturated Fat 1g
  Monounsaturated Fat 6g

○ Cholesterol 0mg

○ Sodium 13mg

○ Carbohydrate 7g
  Fiber 4g

○ Protein 2g

SERVING TIP
For a smooth dip, purée the eggplant in a food processor or blender.

Preparation Time: 35 minutes, plus 1 hour draining, and 1 hour chilling
Serves: 4

SMOKED EGGPLANT & TOMATO SALAD

EGGPLANT IS USUALLY LOW IN CALORIES BUT MAY ABSORB OIL DURING COOKING, SO BROIL OR BAKE THEM TO KEEP THEIR FAT CONTENT LOW. SERVE THIS DISH AS A SIDE DISH OR SPREAD ON BREAD.

1 medium (500g) eggplant, unpeeled
3 medium (350g) tomatoes, skinned, seeded, and chopped
1 small red onion or 4 scallions, finely chopped
1 clove garlic, crushed
2 tbsp extra-virgin olive oil
juice of 1 lemon and 1 tsp grated peel
1–2 red or green chilies, seeded and finely chopped
3 tbsp chopped fresh parsley, mint, or sweet marjoram,
or a combination of the three
freshly ground black pepper, to taste

1 Preheat the oven to maximum. Bake the eggplant whole for 20–25 minutes, until the skin is evenly charred and the flesh is soft. With a sharp knife make a deep cut in the eggplant and place it in a colander to cool slightly.

2 Scoop out the eggplant, leaving the skin intact. Coarsely chop the eggplant and return it to the cleaned colander. Cover, and let it drain for at least 1 hour to remove any bitter juices and excess moisture. (To speed up this process, gently squeeze the eggplant flesh before draining to extract as much moisture as possible.)

3 Finely chop the eggplant until it is almost puréed but still retains some texture. Add the rest of the ingredients, and mix well. Season, and chill for about 1 hour before serving.

VARIATION
Smoked Eggplant and Tahini Salad Omit the tomatoes and oil. Add 4 tablespoons of light tahini mixed with 3 tablespoons of water to the rest of the ingredients in step 3, above. Mix well, season, and chill for about 1 hour before serving.

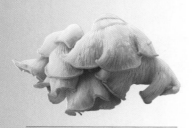

✷ STAR INGREDIENT

Mushrooms, particularly oriental varieties, contain compounds that are reputed to stimulate the immune system and reduce the risk of heart disease.

EACH SERVING PROVIDES:

○ Calories 60

○ Total Fat 4g
  Saturated Fat 1g
  Polyunsaturated Fat 2g
  Monounsaturated Fat 1g

○ Cholesterol 0mg

○ Sodium 100mg

○ Carbohydrate 4g
  Fiber <1g

○ Protein 2g

SERVING TIPS

Serve this delicious, simple dish as an accompaniment to roast or grilled chicken, or as a vegetarian main course with noodles or rice.

Preparation Time: 15 minutes, plus 1–2 hours marinating
Serves: 4

MARINATED & BROILED MUSHROOMS

ASIAN MUSHROOMS – SHIITAKE, OYSTER, OR BLACK TREE

FUNGUS – ARE REPUTED TO REDUCE CHOLESTEROL

LEVELS IN THE BODY, HELPING THE IMMUNE SYSTEM.

6 cups (500g) large oyster mushrooms, trimmed
2 tbsp finely chopped fresh thyme, to garnish

FOR THE MARINADE
1 tbsp toasted sesame oil
1in (2.5cm) piece of fresh ginger, grated
2 shallots, finely chopped
2 cloves garlic, crushed
1 red chili, seeded and finely chopped
4 tbsp rice wine or dry sherry
1–2 tsp honey or sugar

1 Mix together the ingredients for the marinade. Pour the marinade over the mushrooms, and leave to marinate for 1–2 hours, occasionally turning the mushrooms in the liquid.

2 Heat the grill to high, and grill the mushrooms, gill-side up, for 8–10 minutes, occasionally basting them with the marinade, until the mushroom are just cooked and tender.

3 Place the mushrooms in a serving dish. Spoon over the remaining marinade and grill-pan juices, and serve sprinkled with the thyme.

VARIATION
Marinated and Broiled Tofu Replace the mushrooms with 11½oz (350g) tofu, cut into thick slices. Other mushrooms can be used in addition to or instead of the oyster mushrooms. Serve sprinkled with 4 scallions, trimmed and finely shredded, instead of the fresh thyme.

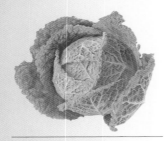

APPLE & CABBAGE SALAD

A REFRESHING AND LIGHT VERSION OF SAUERKRAUT, THIS SWEET AND

SOUR WARM SALAD FEATURES A HEALTHY COMBINATION OF ONIONS,

APPLE, AND CABBAGE. IT CAN BE SERVED ON ITS OWN, WITH PASTA,

OR WITH GRAINS SUCH AS BULGAR, RICE, OR BARLEY.

✶ STAR INGREDIENT
Savoy cabbage is rich in beta-
carotene, an antioxidant
that helps prevent cell damage
by free radicals.

EACH SERVING PROVIDES:

○ Calories 90

○ Total Fat 3g
　Saturated Fat <1g
　Polyunsaturated Fat 1g
　Monounsaturated Fat 1g

○ Cholesterol 0mg

○ Sodium 10mg

○ Carbohydrate 16g
　Fiber 5g

○ Protein 4g

Preparation Time: 30 minutes
Serves: 4

2 onions, finely sliced
6 tbsp apple juice
6 tbsp cider vinegar
1 tsp olive or grapeseed oil
2 tsp black or yellow mustard seeds,
roasted in a dry frying pan
1 small Savoy cabbage, trimmed, cored,
and finely shredded
2 Red Delicious apples, cored, and finely diced
freshly ground black pepper, to taste

1 Place the onions, apple juice, and half the vinegar in a wok or a
large frying pan. Bring to a boil, then reduce the heat, and simmer for
8–10 minutes, until most of the liquid has evaporated. Increase the
heat, add the oil and mustard seeds and cook, stirring continuously,
for 4–5 minutes, until the onions starts to brown.

2 Add the cabbage, apples, and the remaining vinegar. Stir-fry for
2 minutes, or until the cabbage has started to wilt. Season, cover, and
steam over a low heat for 5–8 minutes, until the cabbage is tender
but still retains a slight crunch. Remove the lid, increase the heat, and
boil until most of the liquid has evaporated.

VARIATIONS

Chinese Cabbage and Pear Salad Replace the Savoy cabbage and
apple with Chinese cabbage, finely shredded, and 2 ripe pears, cored
and finely diced.

Pineapple and Cabbage Salad Replace the apple juice with pineapple
juice. Replace the apples with 1 small pineapple, peeled, cored, and
finely chopped.

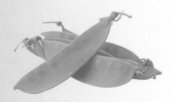

SPRING VEGETABLES WITH ORIENTAL DRESSING

STEAMING IS THE BEST WAY TO PRESERVE THE SWEET FLAVOR

OF VEGETABLES AND TO RETAIN WATER-SOLUBLE VITAMINS THAT

CAN BE LOST DURING BOILING.

*3–4 cups (500g) mixed vegetables, such as broccoli, snow peas,
baby carrots, and zucchini*

FOR THE DRESSING
4 scallions, finely chopped
1in (2.5cm) piece of fresh ginger, finely chopped
1 clove garlic, finely chopped
1 chili, seeded and finely chopped (optional)
4 tbsp mirin
2 tbsp rice wine vinegar or cider vinegar
1 tbsp sesame oil
1 tbsp sesame seeds, roasted in a dry frying pan

1 Steam the vegetables for 4–5 minutes, until just tender.

2 Mix together the ingredients for the dressing, and pour over the warm vegetables. Leave the vegetables to marinate for at least 10 minutes, turning them frequently, to allow the flavors to develop.

VARIATION
Winter Vegetables with Oriental Dressing Replace the spring vegetables with the same quantity of Brussels sprouts, red cabbage, and carrots. Use 1 teaspoon poppy seeds, roasted in a dry frying pan, instead of the sesame seeds.

✶ STAR INGREDIENT
Snow peas contain useful amounts of the antioxidants vitamin C and beta-carotene, as well as fiber, which may lower blood cholesterol levels.

EACH SERVING PROVIDES:

○ Calories 90

○ Total Fat 7g
Saturated Fat 1g
Polyunsaturated Fat 3g
Monounsaturated Fat 2g

○ Cholesterol 0mg

○ Sodium 15mg

○ Carbohydrate 5g
Fiber 3g

○ Protein 4g

BUYING TIP
Mirin is a sweet Japanese wine made from rice. It can be found in oriental shops and some supermarkets.

Preparation Time: 10 minutes, plus 10 minutes marinating
Serves: 4

EACH SERVING PROVIDES:

○ Calories 60

○ Total Fat <1g
   Saturated Fat <1g
   Polyunsaturated Fat <1g
   Monounsaturated Fat <1g

○ Cholesterol 0mg

○ Sodium 6mg

○ Carbohydrate 12g
   Fiber 2g

○ Protein 3g

SERVING TIPS

The grilled vegetables are delicious as an accompaniment to grilled meat or fish, or as a main dish with rice or pasta.

Preparation Time: 25 minutes, plus 1 hour marinating
Serves: 4

MEDITERRANEAN BROILED VEGETABLE SALAD

THIS LOW FAT ADAPTATION OF A FAVORITE MEDITERRANEAN RECIPE FEATURES BRIGHTLY COLORED PEPPERS AND FRESH CITRUS JUICE, BOTH OF WHICH ARE HIGH IN BENEFICIAL ANTIOXIDANTS.

2 red peppers, cored, seeded, and quartered
1 small eggplant, sliced
2 zucchini, sliced
freshly ground black pepper, to taste
fresh basil leaves, to garnish

FOR THE MARINADE
juice of 2 oranges and 1 tsp grated orange peel
juice of 1 lemon
1 tbsp olive oil
1 clove garlic, crushed

1 To make the marinade, mix together the orange juice and peel, lemon juice, olive oil, and garlic in a noncorrosive dish. Mix in the vegetables, and let marinate for about 1 hour. Remove the vegetables from the marinade and drain well. Save the marinade.

2 Heat a griddle and brush it with 1 tablespoon of the marinade. Cook the vegetables for about 3–4 minutes on each side, until just tender and blackened but still crisp, then keep hot.

3 Place the marinade in a small saucepan and bring to a boil until the liquid has reduced to about 3–4 tablespoons. Pour the marinade over the warm vegetables, and mix. Leave to cool to room temperature. Season, and sprinkle with the basil leaves before serving.

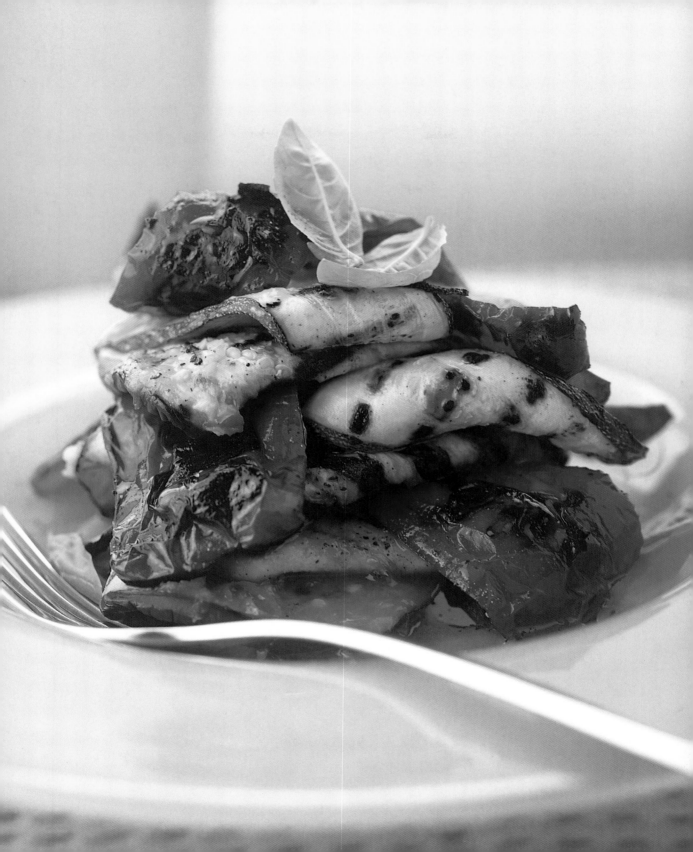

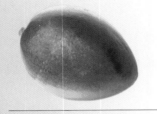

✷ STAR INGREDIENT
Mangoes are a rich source of the antioxidant beta-carotene. It has been shown that those who eat more antioxidant-rich foods are less prone to heart disease.

EACH SERVING PROVIDES:

○ Total Fat <0.5g
  Saturated Fat <0.5g
  Polyunsaturated Fat <0.5g
  Monounsaturated Fat <0.5g

○ Cholesterol 0mg

○ Sodium 36mg

○ Carbohydrate 43g
  Fiber 3g

○ Protein 2g

PREPARATION TIP
You can prepare the sorbet in advance and store it in the freezer for up to a month.

Preparation Time: 15 minutes, plus 4½ hours freezing
Serves: 4

Mango Sorbet

A HEALTHIER, VIRTUALLY FAT-FREE ALTERNATIVE TO ICE CREAM, SORBET MAKES A WONDERFULLY REFRESHING ADDITION TO A MEAL. OTHER SEASONAL FRUITS, SUCH AS SOFT BERRIES, APRICOTS, PEACHES, OR PAPAYA, CAN BE USED INSTEAD OF THE MANGOES IN THIS RECIPE.

2 large mangoes, peeled, pitted, and chopped
juice of 1 lemon
½ cup (100ml) mango juice
2 egg whites
½ cup (100g) sugar
fresh fruits, such as nectarines, berries,
or pineapple, to decorate

1 Place the mangoes, lemon juice, and mango juice in a food processor, and blend until smooth. Transfer the mango purée to a freezer container, cover, and freeze for 45 minutes. Remove the mango purée from the freezer and beat, until almost smooth. Return to the freezer for 45 minutes, or until partly frozen.

2 Place the egg whites in a bowl and whisk to form soft peaks. Continue to whisk while gradually adding half the sugar. Whisk until the mixture forms long peaks, then fold in the remaining sugar.

3 Transfer the mango purée to a food processor. Whisk to break down the ice crystals, and with the machine running, gradually add the egg-white mixture, a tablespoonful at a time. Blend until the mixture turns into a soft slush. Return the mixture to the container, cover, and freeze for 3 hours, or until frozen. Serve decorated with the fresh fruits.

DESSERTS *These low fat desserts will satisfy the sweetest tooth and a wide range of tastes. The mango sorbet and the tangy yogurt ice will refresh the palate, while the sweet polenta pie and the meringue pie are perfect comfort desserts.*

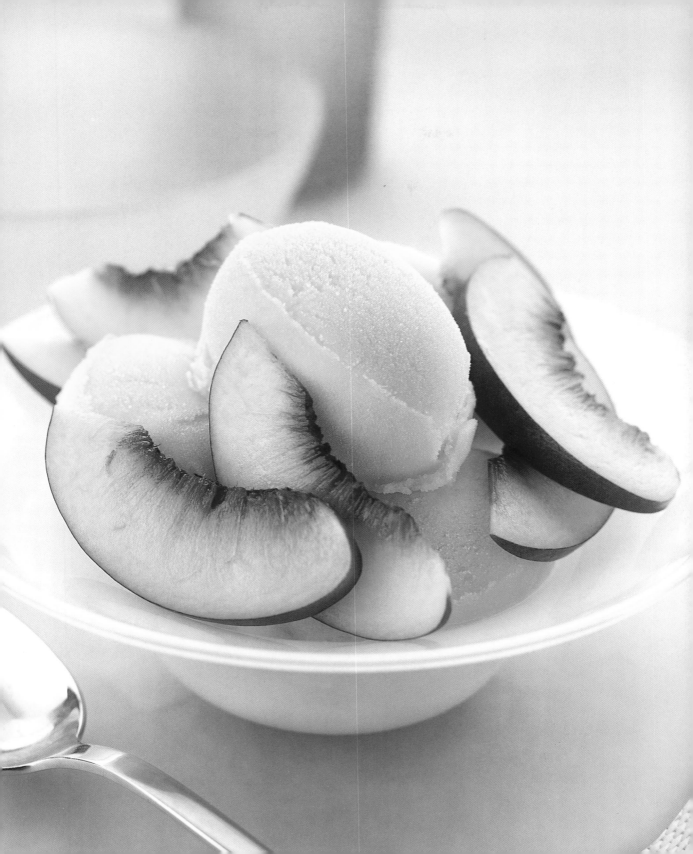

PEAR YOGURT ICE

THIS DELICIOUS AND REFRESHING LOW FAT ICE MAKES
AN IDEAL CONCLUSION TO A SUMMER LUNCH OR DINNER. SOFT
FRUITS, SUCH AS RASPBERRIES, STRAWBERRIES, OR BLACKBERRIES,
ARE PERFECT ALTERNATIVES TO THE PEARS.

6 tbsp water
juice of 1 lemon
1 tbsp honey
1 vanilla bean, halved and seeds scraped out
*2 medium size (400g) ripe pears, peeled,
cored, and quartered*
1 cup (200ml) fat-free plain yogurt
1 egg white
3 tbsp sugar

1 Place the water, lemon juice, honey, and vanilla pod and seeds in a noncorrosive saucepan. Add the pears and bring to a boil. Reduce the heat, cover, and simmer for 20 minutes, or until the pears are tender.

2 Using a slotted spoon, lift out the pears and put them in a food processor. Remove the vanilla bean, then boil the cooking liquid until reduced to 4 tablespoons. Add the liquid to the pears and blend into a smooth purée. Add the yogurt and blend. Spoon the mixture into a freezer container, then leave to cool. Cover, and freeze for 1–1½ hours, until almost frozen, but still soft in the center.

3 Place the egg white in a bowl and whisk to form soft peaks. Continue to whisk, while gradually adding half the sugar, until the mixture forms long peaks, then fold in the remaining sugar.

4 Transfer the semi-frozen yogurt mixture to a food processor. Whisk until soft and smooth. Fold in the egg-white mixture, then transfer to the container and freeze for 1½ hours, or until frozen.

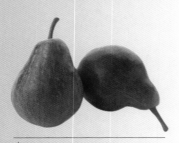

✶ STAR INGREDIENT
Pears are low in fat and contain soluble fiber, vitamin C, and potassium, a combination that helps to lower cholesterol levels and regulate blood pressure.

EACH SERVING PROVIDES:

○ Calories 130

○ Total Fat <0.5g
  Saturated Fat <0.5g
  Polyunsaturated Fat <0.5g
  Monounsaturated Fat <0.5g

○ Cholesterol 0mg

○ Sodium 54mg

○ Carbohydrate 27g
  Fiber 2g

○ Protein 6g

SERVING TIP
Allow frozen desserts to stand at room temperature or in the bottom of the refrigerator for 30 minutes before serving.

Preparation Time: 40 minutes, plus 3 hours freezing
Serves: 4

LAYERED FRUIT & YOGURT MOUSSE

FRESH FRUITS ARE STEEPED IN A CITRUS JUICE AND ORANGE LIQUEUR

MARINADE, AND THEN LAYERED WITH A SOFT AND FLUFFY YOGURT

MOUSSE TO MAKE THIS LIGHT, MELT-IN-THE-MOUTH DESSERT.

juice of 1 lemon and grated peel of ½ lemon
juice of 1 orange and grated peel of ½ orange
3 tbsp orange liqueur or brandy
pulp of 3 passion fruits
4 kiwis, peeled and cut into bite-sized cubes
1 cup (150g) strawberries, hulled and quartered
1 cup (150g) white grapes, halved,
reserving a few, to decorate

FOR THE YOGURT MOUSSE
1 cup (200g) fat-free plain yogurt
1 tbsp lemon juice and ½ tsp grated lemon peel
2 tsp orange flower water, optional
2 egg whites
6 tbsp sugar
½ tsp raspberry vinegar

1 To make the yogurt mousse, beat the yogurt with the lemon juice and grated peel, and the optional orange flower water.

2 Whisk together the egg whites, half the sugar, and the raspberry vinegar to form stiff peaks, then gently fold in the remaining sugar. Fold the egg-white mixture into the yogurt mixture. Line a strainer with a piece of muslin or cheesecloth. Stand the strainer over a bowl, then spoon in the yogurt mixture. Cover, and let it drain in the refrigerator for 3–4 hours, until slightly firm.

3 In a large bowl, mix together the citrus juices and grated peel, orange liqueur, and passion fruit pulp. Add the kiwis, strawberries, and grapes, reserving a few to decorate. Cover, and refrigerate for at least 1 hour. To serve, spoon alternate layers of the marinated fruit and the yogurt mousse in four tall glasses. Decorate with the reserved grapes.

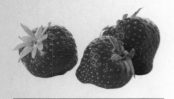

✳ STAR INGREDIENT
Strawberries are rich in fiber and vitamin C and also contain ellagic acid, a reputed protector against the harmful effects of tobacco smoke and pollutants.

EACH SERVING PROVIDES:

○ Calories 220

○ Total Fat <1g
Saturated Fat <0.5g
Polyunsaturated Fat <1g
Monounsaturated Fat <1g

○ Cholesterol 0mg

○ Sodium 77mg

○ Carbohydrate 43g
Fiber 3g

○ Protein 9g

Preparation Time: 15 minutes, plus 3–4 hours draining and 1 hour chilling.
Serves: 4

FIGS WITH MARBLED YOGURT & HONEY SAUCE

FIGS MAKE THE IDEAL LOW FAT DESSERT – SOFT, SWEET, AND
SENSUOUS, WHILE THE HONEY IS A SIMPLE AND DELICIOUS WAY
TO ADD SWEETNESS TO PLAIN YOGURT.

12 ripe figs
1 cup (200g) fat-free plain yogurt, chilled
1–2 tbsp chopped fresh mint, plus sprigs to decorate (optional)
3 tbsp honey

1 Slice each fig into quarters, leaving them attached at the stem end. Arrange the figs on four chilled plates, then press each one gently until they fan out slightly.

2 Spoon the yogurt into a bowl and stir in the mint. Drizzle the honey over the top and carefully fold it in. Add a spoonful of the yogurt sauce to each serving, and decorate with a sprig of mint, if using.

EACH SERVING PROVIDES:

- Calories 160
- Total Fat <1g
  Saturated Fat <0.5g
  Polyunsaturated Fat <1g
  Monounsaturated Fat <1g
- Cholesterol 0mg
- Sodium 43mg
- Carbohydrate 34g
  Fiber 3g
- Protein 8g

Preparation Time: 5 minutes
Serves: 4

MIXED MELON SALAD

1 Cantaloupe melon, seeded
1 small Honeydew melon, seeded
1 tbsp chopped fresh mint
2 tbsp kirsch or apricot liqueur
1 small watermelon, seeded
2 tbsp clear honey

1 With a melon baller, scoop out the flesh from the melons, except the watermelon, into neat balls. Scatter the the mint and sprinkle the kirsch over the melon balls. Cover, and refrigerate for at least 1 hour.

2 Scoop out the watermelon flesh, removing any seeds, and place it in a food processor. Add the honey and blend into a smooth purée. Cover, and refrigerate for at least 1 hour. To serve, divide the watermelon sauce between four plates, then arrange the melon balls on top. Spoon the marinade over the melon and serve.

EACH SERVING PROVIDES:

- Calories 200
- Total Fat 1g
  Saturated Fat <1g
  Polyunsaturated Fat <1g
  Monounsaturated Fat <1g
- Cholesterol 0mg
- Sodium 87mg
- Carbohydrate 43g
  Fiber 3g
- Protein 3g

Preparation Time: 15 minutes, plus 1 hour chilling
Serves: 4

POACHED SPICED PEARS

THESE TENDER, JUICY PEARS POACHED IN A LIGHT

RED WINE ARE HEAVENLY.

2 cups (500ml) full-bodied, fruity red wine
2–3 tbsp honey
4 cardamom pods, crushed
juice and grated peel of 1 lemon
1 small cinnamon stick
1 tsp black peppercorns
4 ripe pears, peeled, with the stems attached
sprigs of fresh mint, to decorate

1 Combine the wine, honey, cardamom, lemon juice and grated peel, cinnamon, and peppercorns in a large, noncorrosive saucepan. Bring to a boil, reduce the heat, skim away any froth, and simmer for 5 minutes.

2 Add the pears and poach gently for 10–15 minutes, until tender. Remove from the heat and let cool. Strain the cooking liquid. Serve the pears in four bowls with a little of the cooking liquid. Decorate each serving with a sprig of mint.

EACH SERVING PROVIDES:

- Calories 100
- Total Fat 0.5g
  Saturated Fat 0g
  Polyunsaturated Fat <0.5g
  Monounsaturated Fat <0.5g
- Cholesterol 0mg
- Sodium 7mg
- Carbohydrate 23g
  Fiber 3g
- Protein 2g

Preparation Time: 25 minutes, plus 10 minutes cooling
Serves: 4

BAKED BANANAS WITH VANILLA

3 tbsp golden raisins
3 tbsp rum
2 tbsp dark brown sugar, or molasses

juice and grated peel of 1 small lemon
4 bananas, thickly sliced
1 vanilla bean, sliced lengthwise into quarters

1 Combine the raisins, rum, sugar, and lemon juice and grated peel in a bowl. Stir in the bananas. Cover, and allow to marinate for 30 minutes.

2 Preheat the oven to 425°F (220°C). Divide the banana mixture between 4 x 8in (20cm) foil rounds, placing it in a small pile in the center of each one. Fold each foil round into a loose package, but do not close the top. Add a quarter of the vanilla bean and a little of the marinating liquid to each package. Close tightly, and bake for 20 minutes, until the bananas have softened. Serve the bananas in their foil packages.

EACH SERVING PROVIDES:

- Calories 180
- Total Fat 0.5g
  Saturated Fat 0g
  Polyunsaturated Fat <0.5g
  Monounsaturated Fat <0.5g
- Cholesterol 0mg
- Sodium 6mg
- Carbohydrate 46g
  Fiber 2g
- Protein 2g

Preparation Time: 30 minutes, plus 30 minutes marinating
Serves: 4

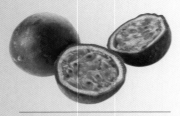

★ STAR INGREDIENTS
Fresh fruits contain beneficial amounts of antioxidants and soluble fiber.

EACH SERVING PROVIDES:

- Calories 120
- Total Fat 2g
  Saturated Fat <1g
  Polyunsaturated Fat <1g
  Monounsaturated Fat 1g
- Cholesterol 0mg
- Sodium 68mg
- Carbohydrate 25g
  Fiber 1g
- Protein 2g

PREPARATION TIP
You can prepare the meringue base in advance and store it in an airtight container for a few days before use.

Preparation Time: 1 hour, 10 minutes, plus 30 minutes cooling
Serves: 6–8

PASSION FRUIT PAVLOVA

THIS IMPRESSIVE, LIGHT, AND INDULGENT DESSERT COULD GRACE THE TABLE OF ANY ELEGANT DINNER PARTY. YET IT IS NOT AS CALORIC AS IT LOOKS – FRESH FRUITS AND ORANGE JUICE ARE EXCELLENT SOURCES OF VITAMIN C AND BETA-CAROTENE.

3 egg whites
1 tsp cream of tartar or 1 tsp raspberry vinegar
½ cup (100g) sugar
2 tsp cornstarch or potato starch

FOR THE TOPPING
pulp of 6 passion fruits
⅔ cup (150ml) fresh orange juice
2 tbsp sugar
2 tbsp cornstarch, dissolved in 2 tbsp orange juice
2 tbsp (30g) low fat unsalted butter
fresh seasonal fruits and mint leaves, to decorate

1 Preheat the oven to 300°F (150°C). Line a baking sheet with waxed paper. In a large bowl, whisk together the egg whites and cream of tartar until they form stiff peaks. Gradually whisk in half the sugar, then fold in the remaining sugar and the cornstarch until the mixture forms long peaks.

2 Spoon the mixture into a 28in (20cm) round on the prepared baking sheet lined with waxed paper. Bake for 1 hour, or until pale gold in color. Turn off the oven, and allow the meringue to cool.

3 To make the topping, place the passion fruit pulp, orange juice, and sugar in a small pan. Bring to a boil, then reduce the heat, and simmer for 15 minutes, or until reduced by half. Add the prepared cornstarch mixture and boil for 1 minute, or until thickened. Remove the mixture from the heat and beat in the butter. Cool the topping.

4 Pour the topping on to the meringue base. Decorate with the fresh fruits and mint leaves, and chill before serving.

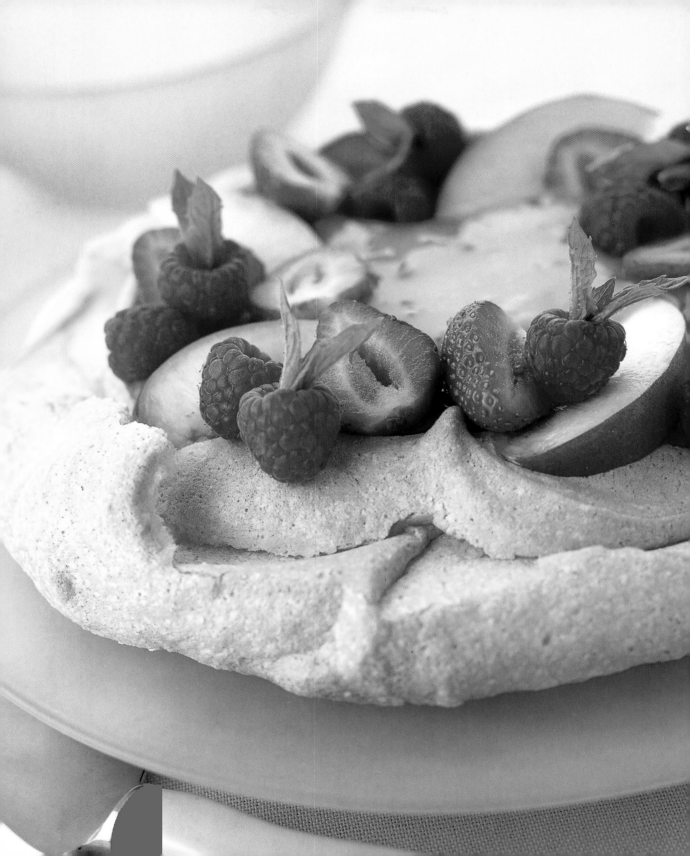

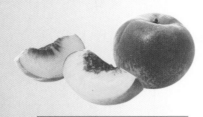

PEACH & GINGER MERINGUE PIE

ANY POACHED FRUITS CAN BE USED IN THIS LOW FAT ALTERNATIVE

TO LEMON MERINGUE PIE, BUT THEY SHOULD BE

FULLY RIPE. SERVE THE PIE WARM OR COLD WITH A SPOONFUL

OF FAT-FREE PLAIN YOGURT.

4 large peaches
⅔ cup (150ml) white wine
2 tbsp lemon juice and the grated peel of 1 lemon
1 stick lemongrass, peeled and halved
1 tbsp honey or sugar
3 egg whites
1 tsp raspberry vinegar
½ cup (100g) sugar
3in (7cm) piece of fresh ginger, finely chopped

1 Steep the peaches in boiling water for 1 minute. Refresh them in cold water, then halve, remove pits, and peel them. Place the wine, lemon juice and grated peel, lemongrass, and honey in a noncorrosive saucepan. Bring to a boil, then reduce the heat, skimming away any froth, and simmer for 5 minutes.

2 Preheat the oven to 400°F (200°C). Return the peaches to the saucepan and poach for 8 minutes, or until just tender. Using a slotted spoon, lift out the peaches, and set aside. Strain the cooking liquid, discarding the grated lemon peel and lemongrass. Return the liquid to the saucepan, then bring to a rapid boil. Boil for 5–6 minutes, until the liquid has reduced and is syrupy and glossy.

3 Whisk together the egg whites and raspberry vinegar, until they form soft peaks, Gradually whisk in half the sugar, then fold in the remaining sugar and the ginger, until the mixture forms long peaks.

4 Arrange the peaches in a 8in (20cm) pie dish. Pour the cooking liquid over the peaches, and spoon the meringue mixture over the top. Bake for 15–20 minutes, until the top is crisp and golden.

✶ STAR INGREDIENT
Peaches are rich in nutrients that are good for the heart, including fiber, potassium, and vitamin C. Like almost all other fruits, they contain no cholesterol.

EACH SERVING PROVIDES:

○ Calories 175

○ Total Fat <0.5g
   Saturated Fat <0.5g
   Polyunsaturated Fat <0.5g
   Monounsaturated Fat <0.5g

○ Cholesterol 0mg

○ Sodium 50mg

○ Carbohydrate 41g
   Fiber 2g

○ Protein 4g

PREPARATION TIP
Canned peaches in natural juice can be used instead of the fresh fruit, if preferred.

Preparation Time: 45 minutes
Serves: 4

APPLE & RASPBERRY COBBLER

IN THIS NEW TAKE ON THE TRADITIONAL COBBLER, FRESH APPLES

AND SOFT BERRIES ARE BAKED UNDER A CRUNCHY GRANOLA

TOPPING OF OATS AND HONEY. A SPOONFUL OF FAT-FREE PLAIN

YOGURT ADDS THE FINISHING TOUCH.

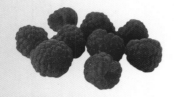

★ STAR INGREDIENT
Raspberries are abundant in the nutrients that are essential for a healthy heart, including vitamins C and E, zinc, potassium, and folate.

EACH SERVING PROVIDES:

○ Calories 220

○ Total Fat 2g
 Saturated Fat <1g
 Polyunsaturated Fat <1g
 Monounsaturated Fat <1g

○ Cholesterol 0mg

○ Sodium 15mg

○ Carbohydrate 48g
 Fiber 4g

○ Protein 4g

PREPARATION TIP
Other fruits, such as plums, rhubarb, blackberries, or peaches, can be used in this dessert.

Preparation Time: 45 minutes
Serves: 6

*6 apples, peeled, cored,
and coarsely chopped*
½ cup (75g) raisins
juice of ½ lemon
*⅔ cup (150ml) dry white wine
or apple juice*
4 cloves
4 tbsp clear honey
1¼ cups (150g) rolled oats
½ cup (100g) raspberries
1 tsp ground cinnamon

❶ Preheat the oven to 425°F (220°C). Place the apples, raisins, lemon juice, wine, cloves, and 1 tablespoon of the honey in a saucepan. Bring to a boil, then reduce the heat, and simmer for 8–10 minutes, or until the apples are just soft.

❷ Remove the apples using a slotted spoon, and place them in a 8in (20cm) pie dish. Bring the cooking liquid to a boil, then boil for 5 minutes, until it has reduced by two-thirds. Pour the liquid over the apples in the pie dish.

❸ In a small saucepan, warm the rest of the honey for 2 minutes, until melted. Mix in the oats and cook for a further 4–5 minutes, until the mixture resembles granola.

❹ Scatter the raspberries over the apples, and cover with an even layer of the oat mixture. Sprinkle with cinnamon and bake for 15 minutes, or until the crumble has browned and is crisp. Serve hot or warm.

MIXED BERRIES WITH SWEET POLENTA PIE

THIS ATTRACTIVE DESSERT FEATURES FRESH BERRIES SERVED

WITH GOLDEN RAISIN POLENTA TRIANGLES. THE TRIANGLES ARE

BEST SERVED WHEN STILL WARM.

2½ cups (300g) mixed berries, such as strawberries, blueberries, and raspberries
4 tbsp Grand Marnier or brandy
juice of 1 orange
powdered sugar, to dust

FOR THE POLENTA PIE
1 cup (250ml) water
juice of 1 lemon
3 tbsp sugar
1 tbsp (15g) low fat unsalted butter
5 tbsp instant polenta or semolina
1 tsp grated lemon peel
½ cup (75g) golden raisins, soaked in a little hot water or orange juice for 20 minutes

1 Sprinkle the berries with the Grand Marnier and orange juice, and allow to marinate for 1 hour.

2 Line a baking sheet with baking paper. To make the polenta, place the water, lemon juice, sugar, and butter in a saucepan, and bring to a boil. Reduce the heat and gradually whisk in the polenta. Cook, stirring frequently, for 5 minutes, until thickened and creamy.

3 Remove from the heat and stir in the grated lemon peel and golden raisins, discarding the soaking liquid. Using a spatula dipped in cold water, spread the polenta into an even, smooth layer, about ½in (1cm) thick, on the prepared baking sheet. Let it cool. Cut the polenta into four triangles. Heat a griddle or skillet and cook the polenta triangles over a medium-high heat for 1–2 minutes on each side, until golden.

4 Transfer the berries with their marinating liquid to four plates, and serve with the polenta. Decorate with a dusting of powdered sugar.

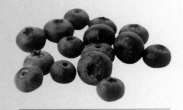

✳ STAR INGREDIENT
Blueberries contain valuable amounts of fiber, vitamin C, and B vitamins. They also feature flavonoids that improve the circulation and aid the body's defenses against infection.

EACH SERVING PROVIDES:

○ Calories 220

○ Total Fat 2g
  Saturated Fat 1g
  Polyunsaturated Fat <1g
  Monounsaturated Fat <1g

○ Cholesterol 5mg

○ Sodium 26mg

○ Carbohydrate 42g
  Fiber 2g

○ Protein 3g

PREPARATION TIP
The polenta triangles can be made the day before and stored in the refrigerator until ready to use.

Preparation Time: 30 minutes, plus 1 hour marinating
Serves: 4

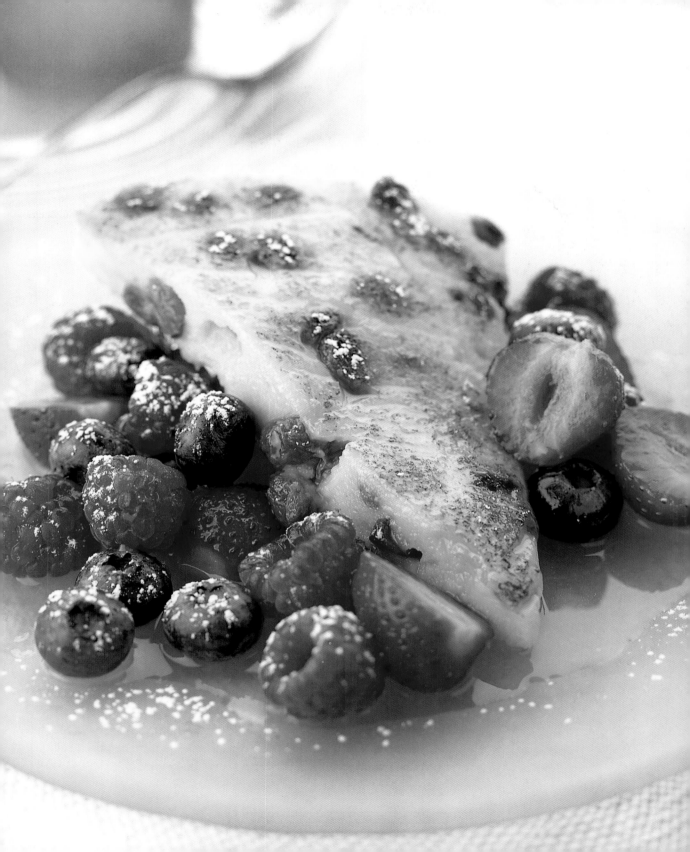

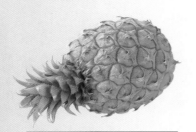

CARAMELIZED PINEAPPLE

NUMEROUS STUDIES HAVE REVEALED THAT BROMELAIN ENZYMES, WHICH ARE FOUND IN PINEAPPLES, AID DIGESTION. THIS SIMPLE DESSERT MAKES THE PERFECT END TO A MEAL, AND IS DELICIOUS WITH A SPOONFUL OF LOW FAT FROMAGE FRAIS.

★ STAR INGREDIENT
Pineapples contain useful amounts of magnesium, zinc, and fiber, as well as antioxidants, which neutralize cell damage by free radicals.

EACH SERVING PROVIDES:

○ Calories 255

○ Total Fat <1g
Saturated Fat 0g
Polyunsaturated Fat <1g
Monounsaturated Fat <1g

○ Cholesterol 0mg

○ Sodium 11mg

○ Carbohydrate 65g
Fiber 4g

○ Protein 2g

PREPARATION TIP
Canned pineapple can be used instead of fresh, but choose fruit that is preserved in natural juice rather than syrup.

Preparation Time: 40 minutes, plus 1 hour chilling
Serves: 4

2 pineapples, peeled and cored
4 tbsp rum or kirsch
2 tbsp sweet white wine, water, or fruit juice
1 vanilla bean, halved lengthways, and seeds scraped out
½ cup (100g) sugar
1 tbsp cornstarch, dissolved in 2 tbsp of wine,
water, or fruit juice
2in (5cm) piece of fresh ginger, finely chopped
1 cup (100g) strawberries, raspberries, or blueberries,
to decorate

1 Slice one of the pineapples into 8 rings, then place the rings in a shallow bowl. Pour 2 tablespoons of the rum over the pineapple, and turn the fruit in the liquid. Cover, and allow to marinate for 30 minutes.

2 Roughly chop the other pineapple. Place the fruit in a noncorrosive saucepan. Add the wine, the vanilla bean and seeds, and ⅓ cup (75g) of the sugar, then stir well. Bring to a boil, then reduce the heat, and simmer for 20 minutes, or until the pineapple is tender.

3 Remove the vanilla bean, then transfer the cooked pineapple to a blender or food processor. Blend for 1–2 minutes, until smooth. Return the pineapple to the pan with the vanilla bean and bring to a boil. Reduce the heat, then stir in the cornstarch mixture. Simmer for a further 1–2 minutes, stirring occasionally, until the pineapple sauce has thickened, then leave to cool. Stir in the ginger and the remaining rum. Refrigerate, covered, for at least 1 hour.

4 Line the broiler rack with foil and preheat the broiler. Place the marinated pineapple rings on the broil rack. Sprinkle with the remaining sugar and broil for 4–5 minutes on each side, or until caramelized. Arrange the pineapple rings on 4 plates, spoon over the sauce and marinade, and decorate each serving with the berries.

PREPARATION TIP
It is important to use the best quality dark chocolate you can find. It should be at least 70 percent cocoa solids.

Preparation Time: 20 minutes, plus 2 hours chilling
Serves: 4

LIGHT CHOCOLATE MOUSSE

THIS IS A HEALTHY ALTERNATIVE TO CHOCOLATE MOUSE FOR SPECIAL OCCASIONS. USE THE BEST CHOCOLATE YOU CAN FIND.

3½oz (100g) 70 percent dark bittersweet chocolate,
broken into chunks
3 egg whites
½ tsp raspberry vinegar
½ cup (100g) sugar
grated peel of 1 orange
strawberries or raspberries, to decorate

1 Put the chocolate in a heat-proof bowl, placed over a saucepan of simmering water. Heat the chocolate until it melts, stirring occasionally.

2 Put the egg whites, raspberry vinegar, and sugar in a heat-proof bowl, placed over a pan of barely simmering water. Whisk the mixture, preferably with an electric hand whisk, for 5–8 minutes, until stiff.

3 Remove the egg-white mixture from the heat, then gently fold in the melted chocolate, making sure that it is thoroughly blended. Pour the mixture into four ramekins. Let them cool, then refrigerate for at least 2 hours. Decorate with strawberries, and serve.

Preparation Time: 30 minutes
Serves: 4

CARAMELIZED RICE PUDDING

4 tbsp sugar
1 tbsp lemon juice
2¼ cups (575ml) water
1 cup (200g) long-grain white rice
1 tbsp (15g) low fat unsalted butter

¼ tsp saffron strands, soaked
in a little warm water
½ cup (75g) raisins
1 tsp grated lemon peel

1 Place the sugar, lemon juice, and 3 tablespoons of the water in a saucepan. Cook over a high heat for 5–6 minutes, until the liquid starts to caramelize. Remove from the heat, then stir in the rice and butter.

2 Stir in the rest of the water, the saffron and its soaking water, and the raisins. Bring to a boil, then reduce the heat. Cover, and simmer for about 20 minutes, until the liquid has been absorbed and the rice is tender. Stir in the grated lemon peel, and serve.

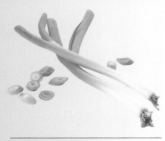

LOW FAT CHINESE DIPPING SAUCE

DIP BAKED TOFU, RAW OR LIGHTLY COOKED VEGETABLES, OR

KEBABS INTO THIS TANGY, SWEET AND SOUR DIPPING SAUCE. IT IS ALSO

DELICIOUS POURED OVER BROILED MEAT OR FISH.

1 tbsp reduced-salt soy sauce
4 tbsp rice vinegar or white wine vinegar
1 clove garlic, finely chopped
1 small carrot, finely grated
½in (1cm) piece of fresh ginger, finely grated
1 tbsp sugar
1 small red chili, seeded and chopped, or ¼–½ tsp chili powder
½ cup (100ml) orange or pineapple juice
1 tsp cornstarch
1 scallion, finely shredded

1 Place the soy sauce, rice vinegar, garlic, carrot, ginger, sugar, and chili in a small, noncorrosive saucepan. Add the orange juice, reserving 1 tablespoon. Bring to a boil, then reduce the heat, and simmer for about 5 minutes, or until slightly thickened.

2 Mix together the cornstarch and reserved orange juice, then stir it into the cooking liquid. Return the mixture to the boil and cook, stirring, until the sauce is thick enough to coat the back of a spoon.

3 Add the shredded scallion and remove from the heat. Serve either hot or at room temperature.

★ STAR INGREDIENT
Scallions contain compounds, such as allicin, that can help to control cholesterol levels, even after a fatty meal.

TOTAL RECIPE PROVIDES:

○ Calories 60

○ Total Fat <0.5g
  Saturated Fat <0.5g
  Polyunsaturated Fat <0.5g
  Monounsaturated Fat <0.5g

○ Cholesterol 0mg

○ Sodium 226mg

○ Carbohydrate 13g
  Fiber 1g

○ Protein 1g

PREPARATION TIP
This sauce can be kept, covered, in the refrigerator for up to 3 days.

Preparation Time: 15 minutes
Makes: ⅔ cup (150ml)

BASICS *This diverse selection of recipes covers*

the techniques that will help to turn the most ordinary dish into a gourmet meal, and unlike many other store-bought sauces, dressings, and stocks, they are all low in fat and salt.

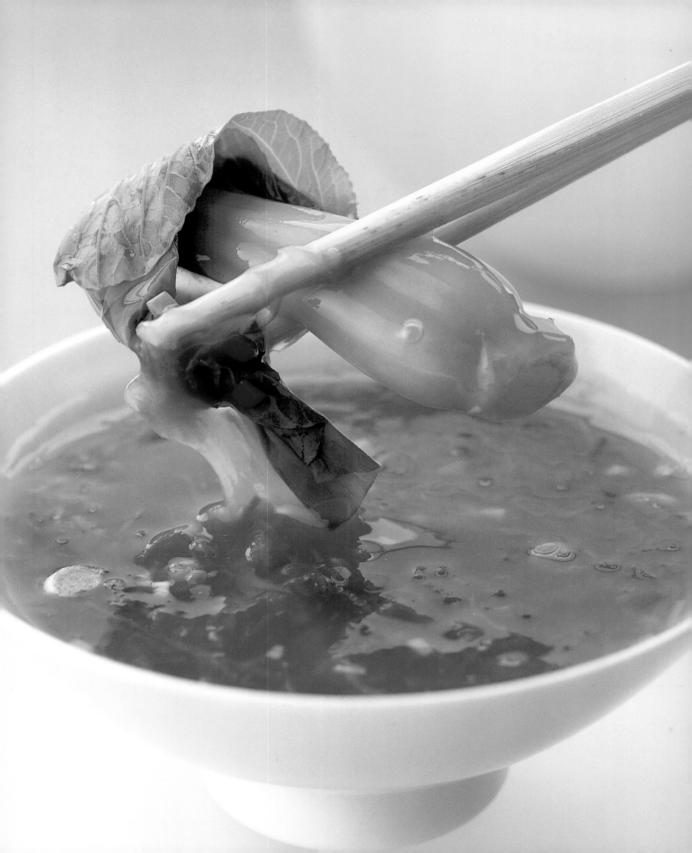

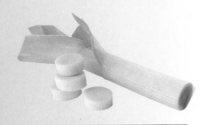

FISH STOCK

2lb (1kg) fish bones, plus heads, and trimmings
1 cup (250ml) dry white wine
6¼ cups (1.5 liters) water
2 leeks, white part only, finely sliced
1 carrot, chopped

1 celery stick, chopped
bouquet garni, made from 2 sprigs of thyme, 2 pieces of green leek leaves, 2 sprigs of parsley, 1 sprig of celery leaves, and 1 bay leaf
10 peppercorns
2–3 thick slices of lemon

1 Wash the fish bones, heads, and trimmings thoroughly in plenty of cold water, then drain well. Place in a large saucepan and add the wine and water. Bring to a boil, skimming away any froth.

2 Add the vegetables, bouquet garni, peppercorns, and lemon. Return to a boil, then reduce the heat, and simmer for 30 minutes, skimming the surface frequently.

3 Strain through a sieve lined with a triple layer of damp cheesecloth or muslin and discard the solids. Allow to cool.

PREPARATION TIPS
To intensify the flavor of the stock include 1 small red mullet, while for a more delicate flavor, use only fish bones.

Preparation Time: 45 minutes
Makes: 6¼ cups (1.5 liters)

PREPARATION TIPS
A chopped apple adds a delicious sweetness to this stock. In addition, ½ cup (75g) okra or 2 tbsp of soaked barley can thicken a stock, giving it a velvety smoothness.

Preparation Time: 45 minutes
Makes: 6¼ cups (1.5 liters)

VEGETABLE STOCK

USE A VARIETY OF VEGETABLES, HERBS, AND SPICES THAT

REFLECT THE SEASON AND EXPERIMENT WITH DIFFERENT TYPES

OF FRESH PRODUCE AND SEASONINGS.

1 large onion, sliced into rings
½ cup (100g) carrots, sliced
3 cloves garlic
½ cup (100g) pumpkin, peeled, seeded, and cubed
3 celery sticks
1 large, ripe tomato, cut into quarters
bouquet garni, made up of 4 sprigs of parsley, 4 sprigs of cilantro, 2 sprigs of thyme, and 2 strips of lemon peel
6¼ cups (1.5 liters) water

Place all the ingredients in a saucepan. Bring to a boil, then reduce the heat, and simmer for 30 minutes. Pour through a strainer lined with a layer of damp cheesecloth or muslin, and discard the solids. Allow to cool.

CHICKEN STOCK

BOUILLON CUBES ARE HIGH IN SALT, SO MAKE YOUR OWN STOCK.

A HOMEMADE STOCK ADDS TEXTURE AND DEPTH TO SOUPS AND

STEWS, AND WHEN REDUCED AND CHILLED, CAN BE USED INSTEAD

OF OIL IN DRESSINGS, MARINADES, OR SALADS.

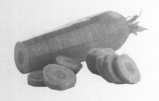

★ STAR INGREDIENT
Carrots provide rich amounts of beta-carotene and vitamin C, which have been shown to reduce blood-cholesterol levels.

PREPARATION TIP
Experiment with different flavorings, such as shallots, fresh ginger, parsley root, and celeriac.

Preparation Time: 2 hours, 45 minutes
Makes: 6¼ cups (1.5 liters)

3–4lb (1.5–2kg) chicken bones, or whole chicken, cut into pieces
1 leek, sliced
1 onion, unpeeled and quartered
4 carrots, coarsely chopped
2 celery sticks, coarsely chopped
bouquet garni, made up of 3 sprigs of thyme, a few celery leaves, 1 bay leaf, and 2–3 strips lemon peel
4 cloves (optional)
1 tsp peppercorns (optional)
1⅓ cups (100g) fresh mushrooms, or 1⅓ cups (5g) dried wild mushrooms, such as porcini (optional)

1 Wash the chicken bones thoroughly in a few changes of water, then drain well. Place the bones in a large saucepan and cover with water. Bring slowly to a boil, then reduce the heat, and simmer for about 30 minutes, skimming away any froth when necessary.

2 Add the vegetables, bouquet garni, cloves, and peppercorns. Continue to simmer the stock for about 1½–2 hours, until it has reduced by about a quarter. Allow it to cool slightly.

3 Strain through a strainer lined with a double layer of damp cheesecloth or muslin, and discard the solids. Allow the liquid to cool. Store refrigerated for up to three days, removing any traces of fat that form on the surface.

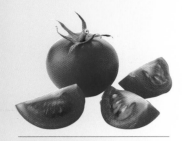

FRESH TOMATO SAUCE

THIS SIMPLE, VIBRANT, FRESH SAUCE CONTAINS A COMBINATION OF TOMATOES, GARLIC, AND ONIONS. IT IS DELICIOUS SERVED OVER PASTA OR RICE, OR AS AN ACCOMPANIMENT TO FISH OR MEAT.

2 onions, chopped
3 cloves garlic, chopped
4 tbsp water
5 tomatoes (1kg) tomatoes, coarsely chopped
1 tsp sugar (optional)
bouquet garni, made up of few sprigs of celery leaves, parsley, oregano, 1 bay leaf, and 1 strip of lemon peel (optional)
1 tbsp olive oil (optional)
salt, to taste

1 Place the onions and garlic in a heavy-based saucepan. Add the water and simmer, stirring frequently, for 5 minutes, or until the water has evaporated and the onion has softened.

2 Add the tomatoes, sugar, and bouquet garni. Simmer, partly-covered, over a very low heat for 1 hour, or until the sauce has thickened. Beat in the oil, if using, and season, then simmer for a few more minutes. Press the sauce through a strainer to remove the bouquet garni and the tomato skins and seeds, and to make a smooth sauce.

VARIATIONS
Spicy Tomato Sauce Add 1–2 red chilies, seeded and chopped, or ½ teaspoon chili powder with the onions in step 1, above.

Tomato and Fennel Sauce For a tomato sauce to serve with fish, add 1 small fennel bulb, finely chopped, with the onions in step 1, above.

Oriental Tomato Sauce Add a 1in (2.5cm) piece of fresh ginger, finely chopped, and 2 star anise with the onions in step 1, above.

✷ STAR INGREDIENT
Tomatoes are a good source of the flavonoid quercetin, as well as the carotene lycopene, which have been shown to reduce the risk of heart disease and strokes.

TOTAL RECIPE PROVIDES:

○ Calories 380

○ Total Fat 20g
Saturated Fat 4g
Polyunsaturated Fat 4g
Monounsaturated Fat 12g

○ Cholesterol 0mg

○ Sodium 96mg

○ Carbohydrate 48g
Fiber 12g

○ Protein 8g

PREPARATION TIP
This sauce can be prepared in advance. Store it in the refrigerator, covered, for up to 3 days.

Preparation Time: 1 hour, 15 minutes
Makes: 2 cups (500ml)

ALMOST FAT-FREE WHITE SAUCE

2 tbsp cornstarch
2 cups (500ml) skim milk
½in (1cm) piece of fresh ginger, grated
1 large (50g) shallot, finely chopped
1 clove garlic, finely chopped (optional)
1 red chili, seeded and finely chopped (optional)

2 tbsp lime or lemon juice
salt and freshly ground white or black pepper, to taste
a little freshly grated nutmeg, to garnish

1 Blend the cornstarch with 2 tablespoons of the milk. Heat the remaining milk in a saucepan, until simmering. Add the cornstarch mixture. Bring to a boil and cook for 1 minute, stirring continuously.

2 Add the ginger, shallots, garlic, and chilli, if using, and the lime juice. Simmer, whisking frequently, for about 15 minutes, or until the sauce is thick enough to coat the back of a spoon, then season. The sauce can be served immediately with a sprinkling of nutmeg or, if a smooth sauce is desired, sieved and reheated.

TOTAL RECIPE PROVIDES:

- ○ Calories 280
- ○ Total Fat 3g
  Saturated Fat 1g
  Polyunsaturated Fat 1g
  Monounsaturated Fat 1g
- ○ Cholesterol 20mg
- ○ Sodium 296mg
- ○ Carbohydrate 56g
  Fiber 2g
- ○ Protein 16g

Preparation Time: 25 minutes
Makes: 2 cups (500ml)

LOW FAT SANDWICH SPREAD

THIS IS A LOW FAT ALTERNATIVE TO BUTTER OR MARGARINE.

FOR A SPREAD THAT IS EVEN LOWER IN FAT, OMIT THE OLIVE OIL

AND USE FAT-FREE CREAM CHEESE.

8oz (250g) low fat or fat-free cream cheese
1 tbsp olive oil
1 small onion, finely grated
1 tsp paprika
¼ tsp chili flakes
1–2 tbsp chopped fresh parsley (optional)
½ tbsp caraway seeds (optional)
salt and freshly ground black pepper, to taste

Beat together the cream cheese and olive oil in a bowl. Add the remaining ingredients and seasoning, then beat well until combined.

1 TABLESPOON PROVIDES:

- ○ Calories 15
- ○ Total Fat <1g
  Saturated Fat <0.5g
  Polyunsaturated Fat <0.5g
  Monounsaturated Fat <0.5g
- ○ Cholesterol 0mg
- ○ Sodium 6mg
- ○ Carbohydrate 1g
  Fiber 0g
- ○ Protein 2g

PREPARATION TIP

The low-fat spread can be kept, covered, in the refrigerator for up to one week.

Preparation Time: 5 minutes
Makes: 1 cup (275g)

1 TABLESPOON PROVIDES:

○ Calories 10

○ Total Fat <1g
　Saturated Fat <1g
　Polyunsaturated Fat <1g
　Monounsaturated Fat <1g

○ Cholesterol 0mg

○ Sodium 1mg

○ Carbohydrate 1g
　Fiber 0g

○ Protein <0.5g

Preparation Time: 15 minutes
Makes: 1 cup (125ml)

1 TABLESPOON PROVIDES:

○ Calories 10

○ Total Fat <0.5g
　Saturated Fat <0.5g
　Polyunsaturated Fat <0.5g
　Monounsaturated Fat <0.5g

○ Cholesterol 0mg

○ Sodium 28mg

○ Carbohydrate 2g
　Fiber <0.5g

○ Protein <0.5g

Preparation Time: 10 minutes
Makes: 1 cup (250ml)

FRUITY SALAD DRESSING

THIS TANGY DRESSING IS RICH IN VITAMIN C AND BETA-CAROTENE.
IT CAN BE SERVED CHILLED AS A SALAD DRESSING, OR HOT
WITH BROILED FISH OR CHICKEN. THE SESAME OIL GIVES IT
A WONDERFUL NUTTY FLAVOR.

1 cup (250ml) orange or pineapple juice
juice of 1 lemon
½in (1cm) piece of fresh ginger, grated
1 tsp mustard powder
1 tbsp dark sesame oil or virgin olive oil
freshly ground black pepper, to taste

1 Place the orange juice, lemon juice, and ginger in a small, non-corrosive saucepan. Bring to a boil, skimming away any froth. Boil the mixture for about 5–8 minutes, or until glossy and syrupy.

2 Remove from the heat, then whisk in the mustard, oil, and seasoning.

MANGO SAUCE

DELICIOUS, VERSATILE, AND VIRTUALLY FAT-FREE,
THIS FRUITY SAUCE GIVES A VIBRANT COLOR AND A CHILI-HOT
FLAVOR TO SALADS, MEAT, OR FISH.

1 small, ripe mango, peeled, pitted, and chopped
juice of 2 limes or 1 lemon
1 tbsp Dijon mustard
1 tsp finely grated lime or lemon peel
1 small chili, seeded and finely chopped (optional)
2 tbsp snipped fresh chives
salt and freshly ground black pepper, to taste

Place the mango flesh and lime juice in a food processor, and blend until smooth. (If the mango is too "stringy" press it through a fine sieve.) Add the remaining ingredients and seasoning, then mix well.

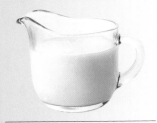

ALMOST FAT-FREE SALAD DRESSING

THIS SMOOTH, SILKY, CREAMY DRESSING IS FULL

OF FLAVOR BUT IT HAS A FRACTION OF THE FAT OF MANY

STORE-BOUGHT COUNTERPARTS.

2 egg yolks
1 tbsp mustard powder
2 tbsp cornstarch
1 tbsp sugar
½ tsp Tabasco
1 cup (250ml) skim milk
⅓ cup (100ml) cider vinegar or white wine vinegar
freshly ground black pepper, to taste

1 Whisk together the egg yolks, mustard, cornstarch, sugar, and Tabasco in a heatproof bowl. Gradually whisk in the milk.

2 Place the bowl over a saucepan of simmering water. Cook, stirring frequently, for 5–8 minutes, until the sauce starts to thicken. Add the vinegar and seasoning, then continue to cook for 3–4 minutes, until smooth and creamy.

VARIATIONS

Fresh Herb Salad Dressing Stir in 3–4 tablespoons chopped fresh mixed herbs, at the end of the cooking time in step 2, above.

Piquant Tomato Dressing Add 2 tablespoons of tomato purée, a clove of garlic, crushed, and ½ teaspoon chili powder with the vinegar in step 2, above.

★ STAR INGREDIENT
Although low in fat, skim milk retains useful amounts of protein, calcium, potassium, zinc, magnesium, folate, and vitamin C.

1 TABLESPOON PROVIDES:

○ Calories 22

○ Total Fat <1g
Saturated Fat <0.5g
Polyunsaturated Fat <0.5g
Monounsaturated Fat <0.5g

○ Cholesterol 21mg

○ Sodium 11mg

○ Carbohydrate 3g
Fiber 0g

○ Protein 1g

PREPARATION TIP
This salad cream will keep for up to a week if stored, covered, in the refrigerator.

Preparation Time: 15 minutes
Makes: 1½ cups (350ml)

INDEX

Page numbers in **bold italics** indicate illustrations. Page numbers followed by an asterisk (*) indicate star ingredients.

NUTRITIONAL DATA

● The nutritional analyses accompanying the recipes are only approximate and are based on data from the food composition tables with additional information about manufactured products, not by direct analysis of the made-up dishes.

● In some cases, the figures for saturated and unsaturated fats do not add up to the total fat figure. This is because the fat total includes other fatty acids and non-fatty acid compounds.

● The symbol "<1g" in the nutritional analyses for the recipes indicates that there is less than 1 gram of the particular nutrient.

● All recipes have been analyzed on the basis of no added salt, unless specified in the recipe.

● Ingredients that are described as "optional" are not included in the nutritional analyses.

ACKNOWLEDGMENTS

Author's acknowledgments: I would like to dedicate this book to Saul, my best taster and washer-upper (and a heart patient). My gratitude also goes to the team: Nicola Graimes, Sue Storey, Jane Suthering, Ian O'Leary, Emma Brogli, and Alison Austin who made this book so delightful and fun to write.

Dorling Kindersley would like to thank Jasmine Challis for the nutritional analyses in the recipe section, Sue Bosanko for the index, Tracy McCord for converting all the recipe metric measurements to American Standard, and Janice Anderson and Stephanie Farrow for editorial assistance. We would also like to thank Lisa Hark, PhD RD, Director of the Nutrition Education and Prevention Program of the University of Pennsylvania Medical Center; Frances Burke, MS, RD, Nutritionist, Cardiac Risk Intervention Program, Philadelphia Heart Institute, Presbyterian Medical Center; David R. Goldmann, MD, Associate Professor of Medicine at the University of Pennsylvania and Senior Deputy Editor of the *Annals of Internal Medicine*; and Diane McCabe, Administrator of the ACP–ASIM Books Program.

Picture credits: the Body Mass Index Chart on page 12 is based on material provided by the Diabetes UK picture library; food photography on pages 12–13 is by Andrew Whittuck.